Examination
Anaesthesia

Examination Anaesthesia

A Guide to the Final FANZCA Examination
2nd edition

Christopher Thomas
BMedSc MBBS FANZCA

Christopher Butler
MBBS FANZCA MPH&TM CertDHM PGDipEcho

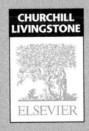

CHURCHILL
LIVINGSTONE

ELSEVIER

Sydney   Edinburgh   London   New York   Philadelphia   St Louis   Toronto

Churchill Livingstone
is an imprint of Elsevier

Elsevier Australia. ACN 001 002 357
(a division of Reed International Books Australia Pty Ltd)
Tower 1, 475 Victoria Avenue, Chatswood, NSW 2067

ELSEVIER

National Library of Australia Cataloguing-in-Publication Data

---

Thomas, Christopher,
Examination anaesthesia: a guide to the final FANZCA examination / Christopher Thomas,
Christopher Butler.

2nd ed.
9780729539470 (pbk.)
Includes index.

Anaesthesia--Australia--Examinations, questions, etc.
Anaesthesia--New Zealand--Examinations, questions, etc.
Anaesthesia--Case studies.

Butler, Christopher Stuart.
Australian and New Zealand College of Anaesthetists.

617.96076

Publisher/Publishing Editor: Sophie Kaliniecki
Developmental Editor: Neli Bryant
Publishing Services Manager: Helena Klijn
Project Coordinator: Natalie Hamad
Edited by Margaret Trudgeon
Proofread by Tim Learner
Cover design by Stan Lamond
Internal design adapted by Lamond Art & Design
Index by Annette Musker
Typeset by TNQ Books & Journals
Moved to Digital Printing 2016

Dedication

To: *Janet, John and Nick Butler*
   Jo Potts
   Abigail and George Thomas

Foreword

Assessment of knowledge in a formal summative examination is a daunting and threatening process for the learner. This is further magnified when the stakes are high, as with the final examination of the Australian and New Zealand College of Anaesthetists (ANZCA). The exam requires the candidates to consider many aspects of life and social structure beyond just acquiring and using knowledge and gaining expertise. Performance at the test requires the candidate to possess knowledge, as well as understand the nature and process of the examination.

There is a relative paucity of information on this process and most is passed down by previous candidates. This book provides the required information and gives guidance on how to prepare for what appears to be a mammoth task for the learner. It will help candidates manage the stress and the emotional rollercoaster of studying for the exam by providing valuable hints and examples. This second edition concentrates solely on the anaesthetic exam, thus eliminating any confusion between the anaesthetic and intensive care exams.

I recommend this book to all ANZCA trainees and International Medical Graduate Specialists in anaesthesia preparing for the final exam. It will also prove useful for educators who take time to teach and prepare potential candidates, as well as those organising courses related to the examination.

Associate Professor Kersi Taraporewalla
MBBS, FFA RACS, FANZCA, MClinEd (UNSW)
Discipline of Anaesthesiology and Critical Care, University of Queensland
Director of Education and Research, Royal Brisbane and Women's Hospital

Contents

Preface

The concept of a guide to approaching a fellowship examination in a medical specialty is not a new one. For as long as examinations have existed, tips and tricks have been passed down from one generation of candidates to the next. The Australian and New Zealand College of Anaesthetists' final fellowship examination is no exception, and much of the inspiration for this book comes from others who have attempted to ease the pain of past examination candidates, most notably Dr Gabriel Marfan, whose remembered preparation and exam experiences from the late 1990s formed the 'Gabe Files', still accessible online. Many other skilled mentors throughout Australasia and the Pacific region have provided invaluable guidance and encouragement for each new generation of anaesthetists approaching the last major hurdle that leads to the FANZCA finish line.

Examination Intensive Care and Anaesthesia was written in 2006, and contained the first incarnation of the volume you now hold. It was the brainchild of Carole Foot and Nikki Blackwell of intensive care fame, who co-opted one of the current authors to provide chapters and information relevant to anaesthesia. The preface of that book contained the prophetic statement: 'As intensive care continues to develop its own identity ... the concept of a combined guide to the examination process for intensivists and anaesthetists will become outmoded.' On 1 January 2010 the College of Intensive Care Medicine was established as an independent entity. By the time this book has been published, *Examination Intensive Care* will also be in production.

The format of the ANZCA final examination has evolved in the last few years, and this update to the exam guide aims to keep pace with those developments. The format, venues, relative weighting and timing of examination components have changed; these are reflected in the overview to the final examination presented in Chapter 1. Useful resources, including new developments on the college website, and strategies for restructuring life around exam preparation are provided in Chapter 2.

Separate chapters based on the major components of the written and clinical exams aim to provide both performance strategies and real examples of the types of questions encountered in the examination. To this end, the last 5 years of written short-answer questions and viva topics have been dissected and sorted under major topic headings. Examples of the types of cases encountered in the medical vivas are given, along with a structured approach to history-taking and examination of such patients, and topics for discussion that candidates might expect in the actual exam.

Despite the culling of the data interpretation viva from the examination format, the ability to interpret common investigations remains a rigorously evaluated attribute through all phases of the examination. The data interpretation section in Chapter 6 aims to provide a structured approach to such investigations, with clinically relevant examples similar to those encountered in the exam.

Finally, a selection of useful references and reviews is provided to serve as the nucleus for candidates' own research and self-directed study.

Those looking for the universal panacea to the final exam will not discover all the answers in this book. Candidates will, however, find advice on how to discover the answers more efficiently for themselves, which is infinitely more useful. The biggest enemy when preparing for the final examination is the inability to effectively manage one's time. It is hoped that the information provided in this volume will both consolidate knowledge and save candidates some of that most precious resource.

We wish candidates all the best in their endeavours.

Chris Thomas
Chris Butler
April 2010

Acknowledgements

Many thanks to Dr Andy Potter, Staff Specialist, Cairns Base Hospital, for his efforts in compiling and categorising many of the review articles presented in Chapter 7.

We also wish to thank the following specialists for their invaluable expertise and insightful input in reviewing the manuscript:

Dr Jim McClean, Staff Specialist, The Ipswich Hospital

Dr Sharon Maconachie, Staff Specialist, The Townsville Hospital

We are grateful to many trainees of recent years for sharing their experiences and insights into the FANZCA training and examination process.

Finally, we wish to acknowledge the efforts of the editorial team at Elsevier in obtaining the relevant permissions from external sources for many of the radiological images which appear in Chapter 6, 'Data interpretation for the ANZCA examination'.

Disclaimer

The authors have taken considerable care in ensuring the accuracy of the information contained in this book. However, the reader is advised to check all information carefully before using it to make management decisions in clinical practice. The authors take no responsibility for any errors (including those of omission) that may be contained herein, nor for any misfortune befalling any individual as the result of action taken using information in this book.

Please note that the opinions expressed in this book are entirely those of the authors, and are in no way intended to reflect or represent those of the Australian and New Zealand College of Anaesthetists; its Joint Faculties past or present; Court of Examiners; Special Interest Groups; subcommittees; other trainees or fellows.

Every attempt has been made to trace and acknowledge copyright, but in some cases this may not have been possible. Apology is made for any accidental infringement, and information enabling us to redress the situation is welcomed.

Abbreviations

A-a	Alveolar–arterial
AAA	Abdominal aortic aneurysm
ABG	Arterial blood gas
ACE	Angiotensin converting enzyme
ACT	Activated coagulation (clotting) time
ADH	Antidiuretic hormone
ADP	Adenosine diphosphate
AF	Atrial fibrillation
AG	Anion gap
AHA	American Heart Association
AHI	Apnoea Hypopnoea Index
AICD	Automatic implanted cardioverter defibrillator
AIDS	Acquired immune deficiency syndrome
ANZCA	Australian and New Zealand College of Anaesthetists
AP	Antero-posterior
aPTT	Activated partial thromboplastin time
ARDS	Acute (adult) respiratory distress syndrome
AS	Aortic stenosis
ASA	American Society of Anesthesiologists
ASD	Atrial septal defect
ATLS	Advanced trauma life support
A-v	Arterio-venous
A-V	Atrio-ventricular
AVA	Aortic valve area
BIS	Bispectral index
BMI	Body mass index
BNP	Type B natriuretic peptide
BP	Blood pressure
BPEG	British Pacing Electrophysiology Group
BSL	Blood sugar (glucose) level
BTPS	Body temperature and pressure saturated with water vapour
BTY	Basic training year
CABG	Coronary artery bypass graft
CAD	Coronary artery disease
CCF	Congestive cardiac failure
CEA	Carotid endarterectomy
CK	Creatine kinase
CNS	Central nervous system
CO_2	Carbon dioxide
COPD	Chronic obstructive pulmonary disease
COX	Cyclo-oxygenase
CPAP	Continuous positive airway pressure
CPR	Cardiopulmonary resuscitation
Cr	Creatinine

CRPS	Complex regional pain syndrome
CSF	Cerebrospinal fluid
CT	Computed tomography
CTR	Cardiothoracic ratio
CVC	Central venous catheter
CXR	Chest X-ray
DC	Direct current
DDAVP	Desmopressin
DIC	Disseminated intravascular coagulation
DKA	Diabetic ketoacidosis
DLCO	Diffusion capacity for carbon monoxide
DLT	Double-lumen tube
ECG	Electrocardiograph
ECT	Electroconvulsive therapy
EDH	Extradural haematoma
EDTA	Ethylenediaminetetraacetic acid
EEG	Electroencephalogram
EF	Ejection fraction
EMAC	Effective Management of Anaesthetic Crises
EMG	Electromyogram
EMLA	Eutectic mixture of local anaesthetics
EMST	Early Management of Severe Trauma
ENT	Ear, Nose and Throat (Otorhinolaryngology)
EOG	Electrooculogram
EPS	Electrophysiological study
ERCP	Endoscopic retrograde cholangiopancreatography
$ETCO_2$	End-tidal carbon dioxide
ETT	Endotracheal tube
FANZCA	Fellowship of the Australian and New Zealand College of Anaesthetists
FBC	Full blood count
$FEF_{25-75\%}$	Forced expiratory flow in middle half of forced vital capacity
FESS	Functional endoscopic sinus surgery
FEV_1	Forced expiratory volume in one second
FiO_2	Fraction of inspired oxygen
FOI	Fibre-optic intubation
FS	Fractional shortening
FVC	Forced vital capacity
GA	General anaesthesia
GCS	Glasgow coma score
GFR	Glomerular filtration rate
Hb	Haemoglobin
HbA1c	Glycosylated haemoglobin
HCO_3	Bicarbonate
HIV	Human Immunodeficiency virus
HOCM	Hypertrophic obstructive cardiomyopathy
HONK	Hyperosmolar non-ketotic coma
HT	Hypertension

IABP	Intra-aortic balloon pump
ICP	Intracranial pressure
ICU	Intensive care unit
IHD	Ischaemic heart disease
INR	International normalised ratio
IV	Intravenous
IVS	Interventricular septum
JVP	Jugular venous pressure
LA	Left atrium
LMA	Laryngeal mask airway
LSCS	Lower (uterine) segment Caesarean section
LV	Left ventricle
LVF	Left ventricular failure
LVIDd	Diastolic diameter of left ventricle
LVIDs	Systolic diameter of left ventricle
LVOT	Left ventricular outflow tract
MA	Maximum amplitude
MCV	Mean corpuscular volume
MCQ	Multiple choice question
MI	Myocardial infarct
MRI	Magnetic resonance imaging
MS	Multiple sclerosis
MV	Mitral valve
MVA	Motor vehicle accident
NASPE	North American Society of Pacing and Electrophysiology
NCA	Nurse controlled analgesia
NEXUS	National Emergency X-Radiography Utilization Study
NIDDM	Non-insulin dependent diabetes mellitus
NNT	Number needed to treat
NOF	Neck of femur
NSAID	Non-steroidal anti-inflammatory drug
NSTEMI	Non ST-elevation myocardial infarct
NYHA	New York Heart Association
O_2	Oxygen
OCP	Oral contraceptive pill
OP	Occipito posterior
ORIF	Open reduction and internal fixation
OSA	Obstructive sleep apnoea
OT	Operating theatre
PA	Postero-anterior
PAC	Pulmonary artery catheter
PACU	Post-anaesthesia care unit
PCA	Patient-controlled analgesia

pCO_2	Partial pressure of carbon dioxide
PDA	Patent ductus arteriosus
PDPH	Post dural puncture headache
PEF	Peak expiratory flow
PEG	Percutaneous endoscopic gastrostomy
PFA	Platelet function analyser
PHT	Pulmonary hypertension
PICC	Peripherally inserted central catheter
PIF	Peak inspiratory flow
PMET	Prevocational medical education and training
pO_2	Partial pressure of oxygen
PONV	Postoperative nausea and vomiting
PPH	Postpartum haemorrhage
PPM	Permanent pacemaker
PR	Pulse rate
PS	Professional standards
PT	Prothrombin time
PTE	Pulmonary thromboembolism
PVD	Peripheral vascular disease
QTc	Corrected QT interval
RA	Right atrium
RDI	Respiratory disturbance index
RERA	Respiratory effort related arousal
REM	Rapid eye movement
RFT	Respiratory function tests
ROTEM	Rotational thromboelastography
RV	Residual volume
RV	Right ventricle
RVSP	Right ventricular systolic pressure
Rx	Treatment
SAH	Subarachnoid haemorrhage
SaO_2	Oxygen saturation
SAQ	Short answer question
SDH	Subdural haematoma
SIADH	Syndrome of inappropriate antidiuretic hormone secretion
SK	Streptokinase
SSS	Sick sinus syndrome
STEMI	ST-elevation myocardial infarct
SVT	Supraventricular tachycardia
T	Tesla
T3	Tri-iodothyronine
T4	Thyroxine
TEG	Thromboelastograph
TIA	Transient ischaemic attack
TLC	Total lung capacity
TOE	Transoesphageal echocardiography
tPA	Tissue plasminogen activator
TSH	Thyroid stimulating hormone
TTE	Transthoracic echocardiography

TURP	Transurethral resection of prostate
TV	Tricuspid valve
U&E	Urea and electrolytes
UK	Urokinase
VAE	Venous air embolism
VF	Ventricular fibrillation
VSD	Ventricular septal defect
VT	Ventricular tachycardia
VTI	Velocity-time integral
WCC	White cell count
WPW	Wolff-Parkinson-White
XR	X-ray

Chapter 1

Overview of the FANZCA final examination

It is better to light a candle than to curse the darkness.
DR CARL SAGAN

FANZCA training scheme

The process of gaining fellowship of the Australian and New Zealand College of Anaesthetists (FANZCA) has undergone numerous changes since the original fellowship process was instituted in 1952. The last major change to the training scheme occurred in 2003 with the introduction of a modular system of training, which requires the trainee to complete 12 formal modules.

Anaesthesia trainees are selected for the training scheme based on a range of selection criteria developed by their individual regional committees. Before being eligible to join the scheme the prospective trainee must have completed two years of Prevocational Medical Education and Training (PMET). This includes one year as an intern and one further year of medical practice, of which no more than 12 months in total can be in anaesthesia, intensive care or pain medicine. The rationale for this requirement is that prospective trainees need to have a solid grounding in general medical practice before entering specialist training.

Prior to commencement of training the college requires that you register as a trainee and provide proof of eligibility. The college also requires that you sign a training agreement that outlines the rights and responsibilities of all parties. During the first two years the trainee undertakes the basic training years ('BTY') 1 and 2. Trainees must complete the primary examination before they can commence advanced training. Theoretically, the primary examination can be attempted at any time after the first year of PMET if a trainee is registered with the college and provides proof of eligibility, but in practice few candidates would have the necessary experience to successfully sit this exam before PMET is completed.

All training time needs to be undertaken in hospitals approved by the college for training of anaesthetists. These hospitals undergo periodic inspection to ensure that the supervision, teaching, case mix and facilities meet a standard acceptable to the college. This aspect is taken very seriously by both the college and the training hospitals, and college recommendations stemming from this process carry considerable weight. All trainees are expected to spend time working in a range of hospitals as part of set rotations. This process ensures that anaesthetists completing ANZCA training have significant breadth of experience.

During the training period formal in-training assessments are carried out (usually on a six-monthly basis) between the trainee and the departmental supervisor of training. This requires the completion of In-Training Assessment Forms that document the progress of professional development and the acquisition of clinical skills.

Candidates wishing to sit for the final examination in anaesthesia need to have completed their two years of basic training, at least one year of advanced training, and passed the primary examination in its entirety. At least four training modules and 24 months of clinical anaesthesia training are also required. These details are laid out in regulation 14 (Examinations in Anaesthesia) and regulation 15 (Training in Anaesthesia), available on the college website (see www. anzca.edu.au/resources/regulations/). The majority of candidates sit the final examination in their second year of advanced vocational training. The prospective trainee is strongly advised to contact the supervisor of training at their hospital for guidance through the process. There is likely to be future change to the nature of the training scheme, as at the time of printing the college was conducting a major review of the curriculum.

Once candidates have passed the final examination they must submit a satisfactory formal project and complete the Early Management of Severe Trauma (EMST) or Effective Management of Anaesthetic Crises (EMAC) course to satisfy the requirements of fellowship. Ideally, these requirements are completed between the primary and final examinations. Candidates also need to successfully complete all 12 curriculum modules and the full 60 months of clinical training, of which at least 33 months are required in clinical anaesthesia and at least three months in intensive care medicine.

Once you are admitted to fellowship you are entitled to be presented at a college ceremony, which is held as part of the college annual scientific meeting each year.

Format of the final examination

Timing and location

The final examination is held twice a year, with the written paper and medical viva section usually held in March or early April, and again in July or early August. The anaesthesia vivas are held six to eight weeks after the written paper. The closing date to apply for the exam is approximately two months prior to the written section. The closing date and application to sit the examination are available on the college website. This deadline is strictly upheld by the college. Applications to sit must be accompanied by the examination fee (A$4255 as of early 2010). Although this fee is a significant cost to the candidate, the running of the exam is an expensive process for the college. The examiners themselves are not paid for their services and they invest considerable time in the process.

Candidates who have applied to sit can withdraw from the exam not less than 56 days before the date of the exam and receive a refund of examination fees by formally notifying the assessments unit of the college in writing. If this application occurs ten days or less before the day of the written examination a 10% (= A$425.50) administration fee will be incurred. If a candidate withdraws from the exam less than two days before the written exam no refund will apply, unless there are exceptional circumstances (which must be notified to the college with supporting documentation).

The written exam is currently held in Sydney, Melbourne, Brisbane, Adelaide, Perth, Auckland and Hong Kong. The medical vivas are held in the same cities on the following day.

The anaesthesia vivas are usually held in Melbourne in May and Sydney in September/October, but dates and venues vary slightly from year to year. In recent times the vivas have been held in large function venues instead of at the college, due to the number of candidates taking the exam. The Sydney exam is generally held at Randwick Racecourse, and the Melbourne exam at the Melbourne Convention and Exhibition Centre. Candidates present for the anaesthesia vivas if they have passed at least one part of the short answer, multiple choice or medical vivas. Candidates are notified as soon as possible that they are to attend the anaesthesia vivas, usually with three to four weeks' notice. This delay in notification is due to the time required by the college and the examiners to distribute, mark and return the short answer papers.

The written examination

The written examination is conducted in two sessions held on the same day (usually a Friday). The morning session consists of 150 multiple choice questions to be completed in 2.5 hours (with 10 minutes for perusal). The afternoon session comprises 15 short answer questions to be completed in 2.5 hours (also with 10 minutes for perusal). During the perusal time candidates are not allowed to make any marks on the answer papers.

Overseas specialists seeking Australian qualifications may be granted an exemption from the multiple choice component of the exam. However, as the multiple choice paper historically has a higher pass rate than the short answer paper, many exempted candidates still elect to sit the whole exam as this is perceived to increase their overall chance of passing. There is no clear consensus or proof that this is in fact the case.

Multiple choice paper

The multiple choice component is worth 20% of the final examination mark. It encompasses all areas of modern anaesthesia (and their minutiae), clinical pharmacology in its entirety, and all of general medicine and its subspecialties. It is also the component of the exam where primary examination material is most likely to be tested. Although this scope of content may appear daunting, all of the questions are in some way based on a part of the modular curriculum.

All questions are currently 'type A', where there is a single correct answer from within five alternatives. The question has a stem that defines the task, usually as part of a sentence, and options that complete the sentence. There are a number of 'black banks' of questions available that are produced from the remembered questions supplied by past candidates. The most useful of these is available at www.anaesthesiamcq.com, which provides several of sets of multiple choice questions, as well as a range of web-based tutorials. The college also now publishes the actual questions after a three-year delay (www.anzca.edu.au/trainees/atp/final-examination/examination-reports/final-examination-reports.html). These are well worth studying in considerable detail, as they not only allow for reading around the topics being examined, but also show the differences between the actual questions and the versions remembered in the black banks.

The multiple choice exam is comprised of different types of questions (although this is not always obvious to the candidate). Most important are the marker questions, which have been asked before and are known to be good discriminators (i.e. the good candidates get them right and the weaker candidates get them wrong). By definition, these will have been asked before and may be included in the list of questions published by the college. Other (non-marker) repeat questions also appear that may have occurred in recent exams. There will also be a selection of new questions.

Each member of the panel of examiners is expected to produce a number of multiple choice questions per year. The process of writing a multiple choice question is difficult and time-consuming for the examiner. It is very likely that the examiners will think of questions to write while they are marking short answer questions or preparing viva questions. This means that it is also useful to look at the subject matter in recent short answer papers and vivas, as they may well have spawned a mutant offspring in the multiple choice questions.

Many new questions appear to be sourced from current developments in knowledge as expressed in journals and scientific meetings, and periodicals such as *Australasian Anaesthesia*.

The quality of each question in any particular multiple choice paper is analysed for its difficulty and its ability to discriminate between candidates as judged by its performance against the marker questions. Negatively discriminating questions may be dropped from the analysis of the results on the basis that they may have been poorly written, are confusing, or the answer could be wrong. It must be remembered that as medical knowledge evolves, questions that were previously good may become ambiguous, especially to the better candidate with a greater depth of knowledge.

There is no negative marking in the multiple choice examination, so it is important that you attempt every question. It is also important to check that your answer corresponds with the correct number on the answer sheet. This section is marked by computer and a sequence error on the answer sheet is disastrous.

Short answer paper

The short answer component is worth 20% of the final examination mark. It also covers a broad range of topics. There are 15 questions to be answered in 150 minutes, so it is critical to master the skill of discipline in adhering to time limits. The ability to write a good response to the short answer question is acquired through practice, and candidates are well advised to do this repeatedly under mock exam conditions. Historically this is the component of the exam in which candidates perform the worst (see Table 1.1). The college obviously believes that this section is both important and has been underrated by past candidates, hence the recent (2009) increase in the relative value of the marks attached to it.

More so than any other section, the short answer questions test the ability of candidates to synthesise a large amount of information into a logical structured form in a short amount of time. All of the short answer questions from recent examinations are available on the college website. It is well worth studying the subject matter of past questions in detail, especially if they have been poorly answered. Remember, the processes of short answer question marking and preparation may inspire examiners to repeat such questions in a later examination, particularly during anaesthesia vivas or as multiple choice questions.

TABLE 1.1 Percentage of candidates passing final examination components, 2005–09

Year	Multiple choice questions	Short answer questions	Anaesthesia vivas	Medical vivas
2005 (1)	78	44	90	87
2005 (2)	84	62	94	83
2006 (1)	88	62	94	89
2006 (2)	79	42	92	80
2007 (1)	92	52	90	89
2007 (2)	91	45	87	75
2008 (1)	84	47	82	73
2008 (2)	85	50	80	69
2009 (1)	67	30	90	76
2009 (2)	77	30	75	66

Each question in the short answer paper needs to be answered in a separate examination booklet. This is because each question is sent to a separate examiner for marking, i.e. one examiner will mark the efforts of all 200-odd candidates on a particular question. It is also important to write as legibly as possible. Although the marker will go to considerable efforts to be fair and interpret the well-intentioned efforts of a candidate, if the paper cannot be read then marks cannot be awarded.

It is important to write something on the paper for each question, no matter how little you know about the topic. It is fairly easy to gain 2 or 3 marks for a limited answer (compared to 0 marks for no response). Improving a good answer from 5 or 6 marks to an excellent one (greater than 7 or 8 marks) for a question you believe you know a lot about is actually far more difficult and time consuming. Not leaving any question blank will greatly increase your chances of passing.

The written examination is discussed further in Chapter 3.

The clinical examination

Medical vivas

The medical vivas comprise 12% of the final examination mark. The aim of the medical vivas is to assess the ability of the candidate to take a focused history and examination, interpret investigations in relation to the patient, assess the functional state of the patient and discuss the implications of their medical condition for anaesthesia and surgery. This is the set of skills required to undertake a detailed preoperative assessment. The medical viva is the only time during the entire examination process that you are directly observed by an examiner interacting with an actual patient.

This component of the exam underwent two significant changes in 2008. Prior to this there were three medical vivas held in conjunction with the anaesthesia vivas, two with patient history and examination, and one investigations viva, each of 15 minutes duration.

Firstly, the specific investigations viva was dropped, and the other two medical vivas extended to 18 minutes. This allows for a bit more time to be spent with the patient, and also increases the likelihood of investigations being incorporated in a discussion relating to the actual patient.

Secondly, the medical vivas are now held the day following the written exam, and in the same city. This change has arisen from the logistical difficulties associated with assembling enough suitable patients in one venue for the ever-increasing number of candidates. The medical vivas are thus spread over several centres, vastly increasing the pool of quality patients available for the examination. It is also possible for the examiners to obtain patient details sooner, which helps in the preparation of questions and the smooth running of the viva. You are also more likely to meet an examiner who you know in the medical viva, as most of the examiners will be from your regional centre.

The disadvantage of this latter change is that candidates who live outside the examination centres need to make two trips for the exam, necessitating extra expenses and disruption. It also means that candidates need to prepare for the medical vivas earlier, and not ignore them until after the written exam, as they tended to do in the past.

Each candidate is given two minutes perusal time prior to the viva, when they are able to read the patient's introductory details and what is expected of them in the viva. Often you will be supplied with a list of a patient's medications (as this saves time in the history-taking component). Upon entering the room the examiner will verify your candidate number, introduce you to the patient and repeat the task required, which will involve a focused history and examination. You are expected to spend between eight and nine minutes with the patient; the examiner will give a time reminder towards the end of this time. Following your time with the patient you are expected to wash your hands and present your findings. The examiner is present for the whole time and will be marking candidates on their performance throughout.

The criteria for marking include the history-taking, examination skills, communication skills, clinical judgement, synthesis of findings, professionalism, organisation, efficiency and the examiner's overall impression. Most of the patients are old hands at the examination process and are well versed in their condition. They are likely to be much more forthcoming with information if you treat them nicely.

Each medical viva is worth 6% of the total marks in the exam. There is no requirement to pass both medical vivas to pass the section, but simply to get more than 50% in total to pass this section.

In years gone by there were two examiners for the medical vivas – one anaesthetist and one physician. Now the examination is undertaken by one anaesthetist only. If there is a second person in the room they will be observing the performance of the examiner.

The medical vivas are discussed further in Chapter 4.

Anaesthesia vivas

The anaesthesia vivas comprise 48% of the final examination mark. There are eight anaesthesia vivas, each of 15 minutes duration, held six to eight weeks after the written exam. Candidates are divided into two groups, with each group completing their vivas on a single day. Four vivas are held in the morning session and four in the afternoon. Candidates are advised in writing by the college exactly what time they must attend the examination venue.

At the commencement of each session candidates will be addressed by the chair of the court of examiners and presented with a coloured card (the colour denotes your rotation of four stations). This card lists the order in which the vivas will be attempted. Those candidates with the same coloured card will rotate around the same examiners. All the candidates being examined on the same day will be presented with the same scenarios for the anaesthesia vivas.

Each anaesthesia viva is preceded by two minutes preparation time, the start of which is signalled by a bell. The clinical scenario and opening question are printed on a piece of paper attached to the wall opposite the examination booth. This question may well be accompanied by an investigation relating to the case. Candidates may make notes if they wish. After two minutes another bell sounds for the candidate to enter the examination booth and greet the examiner. The examiners will introduce themselves and check your candidate number. Save time by showing it to them without them asking to see it. Another copy of the clinical scenario (and accompanying investigation, if present) will be attached to the desk, and the examiner will begin by restating the opening question. At the conclusion of the viva a bell sounds (which also marks the start of the next perusal period), and candidates move immediately to the next station where the process is repeated.

The rotation of four vivas usually includes a fifth rest station. Candidates from the other rotations who are sitting the vivas in the same order converge at the rest station (everyone will have a different coloured card with the vivas listed in the same order). There is normally a selection of light refreshments, with tea and coffee provided. Once the group has completed a set of four vivas, they will be quarantined from the other group that is yet to complete the set.

Each of the eight anaesthesia vivas will involve a cross-table discussion of a clinical scenario, often with the interpretation of investigations relating to the case, and usually including a component of crisis management. Each viva will generally run through three major key issues. There will be a different examiner for each of the eight anaesthesia vivas. The college attempts to avoid candidates encountering an examiner they have met in the medical vivas, but sometimes this is impossible to achieve.

There is no requirement to pass any minimum number of vivas to pass the examination, but you need to get at least 50% to pass the anaesthesia vivas and hence the examination overall.

The anaesthesia vivas are discussed in greater detail in Chapter 5.

Marking components of the final examination

As mentioned above, the 100 marks in the final examination are distributed as follows:

Multiple choice questions	20
Short answer questions	20
Medical vivas	12
Anaesthesia vivas	48

To pass the final examination, candidates need to score at least 50% for the entire exam, pass the anaesthesia viva component, and pass at least one other component of the exam. Table 1.1 (see page 5) outlines the pass rates for the various components of the examination in recent years.

The results are announced that evening for those candidates examined that day, as well as being posted on the college website. The successful candidates are then presented to the court of examiners and invited for a drink. Family members of the successful candidates are also welcome to attend this event.

Unsuccessful candidates are sent a breakdown of their marks by post after the examination. The college has also instituted a process of feedback interviews for unsuccessful candidates to assist in their preparation for further attempts.

The candidate who achieves the best result at each final exam may be awarded the Cecil Gray Prize at the discretion of the college. The decision is announced several weeks after the examination and the winner is usually contacted by telephone and post. The prize is a great honour and is presented at a major college meeting. In addition, a small number of candidates may be chosen to receive merit awards, reflecting their outstanding performance at the examination. These candidates receive a special letter of commendation from the college, and the list of recipients is published in the *ANZCA Bulletin*.

Chapter 2

Preparation for the final examination

Alcohol is the anaesthesia by which we endure the operation of life.
  GEORGE BERNARD SHAW

Resources

The scope of the final examination in anaesthesia is formidable. It covers the application of the basic sciences (as tested in the primary examination), as well as a suitable grounding in all the anaesthetic subspecialty areas. As an exit examination it seeks to determine whether a candidate can safely assess and manage any clinical problem that may confront them in their daily work as a consultant anaesthetist.

Equally daunting is the volume of material from which knowledge can be drawn. Given the limited amount of preparation time available, candidates need an efficient method of acquiring facts and an understanding of all important topics. Textbooks and journals are still the most useful sources of information, but internet-based resources are increasing in number, breadth of subject matter and usefulness. However, when retrieving information online be mindful to question the scientific validity and academic integrity of all sources.

Always remember the value of human resources. Enlist the help not only of your colleagues sitting the exam, but also of your supervisor of training and individual module supervisors, other specialists and registrars from anaesthesia, medicine and intensive care, and, most importantly, recent successful examination candidates. All of these people have knowledge and skills that are invaluable in successfully guiding you to the end of the training and examination process.

The college website
The college website (www.anzca.edu.au) is a vast resource, a major component of which is essential information on the training process, available at www.anzca.edu.au/trainees/. Useful features include the ability to access your training profile online (which contains all of the relevant information kept by the college on your training to date), a complete description of the training and examination processes, and specific learning resources.

9

Curriculum

The 12 curriculum modules aim to break down the vast training experience into manageable chunks. All twelve modules must be completed, verified by the module supervisor and/or supervisor of training in your hospital, and the relevant documentation submitted to the college. The modules which need to be completed in 60 months are:

Module 1   Introduction to Anaesthesia and Pain Management
Module 2   Professional Attributes
Module 3   Anaesthesia for Major and Emergency Surgery
Module 4   Obstetric Anaesthesia and Analgesia
Module 5   Anaesthesia for Cardiac, Thoracic and Vascular Surgery
Module 6   Neuroanaesthesia
Module 7   Anaesthesia for ENT, Eye, Dental and Maxillofacial Surgery
Module 8   Paediatric Anaesthesia
Module 9   Intensive Care
Module 10 Pain Medicine – Advanced Module
Module 11 Education and Scientific Enquiry
Module 12 Professional Practice

Not only do the modules dictate your training time, they also form a useful framework around which to plan your study for the examination. As well as training aims and learning objectives, each curriculum module lists in great detail specific topics that you need to gain knowledge of, and the relevant clinical skills you need to acquire. These topics form a useful checklist for study purposes. Analysis of the detailed content of the modules is beyond the scope of this book, but the modules in their entirety can be found at www.anzca.edu.au/trainees/atp/curriculum.

Past papers

Previous examination papers and examination reports are available on the college website and provide an invaluable insight into the scope of knowledge and standard required to pass the final examination.

The publishing of entire multiple choice papers is a recent innovation by the college. These carry a vintage of three years (presumably to afford some protection to recent, new and marker questions that may be repeated in consecutive exams) and are an incredibly useful preparation tool. The examination report for each paper also lists a distribution of topics covered by the questions (which remains relatively constant between exams). This may help candidates apportion their study time appropriately.

The short answer question paper is listed in its entirety in each report, along with a detailed analysis of the information required to pass each question. In recent years the manner in which examiners have apportioned their marks for some questions has been included. In some cases a complete model answer for a topic is provided. Poor approaches to a question and candidate misconceptions are also highlighted.

The examination reports summarise the overall performance of candidates in the medical viva section and the manner in which marks are allocated (which is constant from year to year). The examination report from the second sitting of 2009 set a precedent by listing the primary medical conditions encountered by candidates in the medical vivas.

The final section of the examination report lists all 16 introductory scenarios of the anaesthesia vivas. This section has also recently included the aims of each viva, giving candidates a new insight into the flow of a viva and the subsequent topics asked.

It is difficult to imagine how the college could more directly indicate to candidates the scope and standard required of them in the final examination than through these reports. Candidates ignore these at their peril.

Professional documents

A commonly forgotten but extremely useful resource available on the college website is the section devoted to the professional documents of the college. Not only do these contain useful summaries of topics of major importance, but each one lends itself to the creation of a short answer question or viva topic. A thorough knowledge of their contents is likely to stand a candidate in good stead as they address all important points and a wide range of detail on a particular topic. Examination reports repeatedly highlight the need to be familiar with the more important of these, and those listed below may be of particular interest:

Professional standards
- PS3: Guidelines for the Management of Major Regional Analgesia
- PS4: Recommendations for the Post-Anaesthesia Recovery Room
- PS6: The Anaesthesia Record. Recommendations on the Recording of an Episode of Anaesthesia Care
- PS7: Recommendations on the Pre-Anaesthesia Consultation
- PS8: Guidelines on the Assistant for the Anaesthetist
- PS9: Guidelines on Sedation and/or Analgesia for Diagnostic and Interventional Medical or Surgical Procedures
- PS10: The Handover of Responsibility during an Anaesthetic
- PS12: Statement on Smoking as Related to the Perioperative Period
- PS15: Recommendations for the Perioperative Care of Patients Selected for Day Care Surgery
- PS16: Statement on the Standards of Practice of a Specialist Anaesthetist
- PS18: Recommendations on Monitoring During Anaesthesia
- PS19: Recommendations on Monitored Care by an Anaesthetist
- PS20: Recommendations on Responsibilities of the Anaesthetist in the Post-Anaesthesia Period
- PS21: Guidelines on Conscious Sedation for Dental Procedures in Australia
- PS26: Guidelines on Consent for Anaesthesia or Sedation
- PS28: Guidelines on Infection Control in Anaesthesia
- PS29: Statement on Anaesthesia Care of Children in Healthcare Facilities Without Dedicated Paediatric Facilities
- PS31: Recommendations on Checking Anaesthesia Delivery Systems
- PS37: Statement on Local Anaesthesia and Allied Health Practitioners
- PS38: Statement Relating to the Relief of Pain and Suffering and End of Life Decision
- PS39: Minimum Standards for Intrahospital Transport of Critically Ill Patients
- PS41: Guidelines on Acute Pain Management
- PS43: Statement on Fatigue and the Anaesthetist
- PS49: Guidelines on the Health of Specialists and Trainees
- PS50: Recommendations on Practice Re-entry for a Specialist Anaesthetist
- PS51: Guidelines for the Safe Administration of Injectable Drugs in Anaesthesia

Technical
- T1: Recommendations on Minimum Facilities for Safe Administration of Anaesthesia in Operating Suites and Other Anaesthetising Locations
- T3: Minimum Safety Requirements for Anaesthetic Machines for Clinical Practice

Training
- TE5: Policy for Supervisors of Training in Anaesthesia
- TE6: Guidelines on The Duties of an Anaesthetist
- TE14: Policy for the In-training Assessment of Trainees in Anaesthesia

Final examination preparation resource

Towards the end of 2009 the college uploaded the Final Examination Preparation Online Resource, created by Dr Alex Konstantatos, which comprises an indexed and linked series of video clips. These videos explain each of the many facets of the exam and contain many useful study, time management and performance pointers. There is also a series of simulated anaesthesia vivas conducted by actual examiners, illustrating a range of viva technique problems. There are examples of good viva technique and also some candidate attitudes and approaches that are best avoided. Also of interest are the perspectives of a past chairman of the final examination court. Considerable effort has obviously gone into the professional production of this resource, which is well worth looking at prior to preparing for the exam, as well as immediately before sitting. It can be found at www.anzca.edu.au/edu/projects/distance-education/fepor/.

Textbooks

Major textbooks of anaesthesia provide a solid foundation of knowledge when you are preparing for the examination, and a source for further reading around specific topics. Which of these textbooks a candidate chooses as a primary reference is a matter of personal preference, and you should look at a range of texts to see which you prefer. Some useful reference texts are listed below. All of these should be available for loan from the college library.

Airway management

Hagberg, CA, ed. Benumof's airway management: principles and practice. 2nd edn. Philadelphia: Mosby Elsevier, 2007.

Hung OR, Murphy MF, eds. Management of the difficult and failed airway. New York: McGraw-Hill Medical, 2008.

Kovacs G, Law JA. Airway management in emergencies. New York: McGraw-Hill, 2008.

Orebaugh SL. Atlas of airway management: techniques and tools. Philadelphia: Lippincott Williams and Wilkins, 2007.

Walls RM, ed. Manual of emergency airway management. 3rd edn. Philadelphia: Lippincott Williams and Wilkins, 2008.

Anatomy

Ellis H, Feldman S. Anatomy for anaesthetists. 8th edn. Carlton: Blackwell Publishing, 2004.

Erdmann AG. Concise anatomy for anaesthesia. London: Greenwich Medical Media, 2002.

Applied physiology and pharmacology

Brunton LL, ed. Goodman and Gilman's the pharmacological basis of therapeutics. 11th edn. New York: McGraw-Hill, 2006.

Peck TE, Hill SA, Williams M. Pharmacology for anaesthesia and intensive care. 3rd edn. Cambridge: Cambridge University Press, 2008.

Power I, Kam P. Principles of physiology for the anaesthetist. 2nd edn. London: Arnold, 2008.

Cardiothoracic anaesthesia

Gravlee GP, Davis RF, Kurusz M, Utley JR, eds. Cardiopulmonary bypass: principles and practice. 2nd edn. Philadelphia: Lippincott Williams and Wilkins, 2000.

Hensley FA, Martin DE, Gravlee GP, eds. A practical approach to cardiac anesthesia. 4th edn. Philadelphia: Wolters Kluwer – Lippincott Williams and Wilkins, 2008.

Kaplan JA, Reich DL, Lake CL, Konstadt SN, eds. Kaplan's cardiac anesthesia. 5th edn. Philadelphia: Elsevier Saunders, 2006.

Mackay J, Arrowsmith J, eds. Core topics in cardiac anaesthesia. Great Britain: Greenwich Medical Media, 2004.

Sidebotham D, Merry A, Legget M, eds. Practical perioperative transoesophageal echocardiography. Butterworth-Heinemann Elsevier, 2003.

Youngberg JA, Lake CL, Roizen MF, Wilson RS, eds. Cardiac, vascular, and thoracic anesthesia. New York: Churchill Livingstone, 2000.

Complications

Lobato EB, Gravenstein N, Kirby RR, eds. Complications in anesthesiology. Philadelphia: Wolters Kluwer – Lippincott Williams and Wilkins, 2008.

Neal JM, Rathnell JP, eds. Complications in regional anesthesia and pain medicine. Philadelphia: Elsevier Saunders, 2007.

Crisis management

Allman KG, McIndoe AK, Wilson IH, eds. Emergencies in anaesthesia. 2nd edn. Oxford: Oxford University Press, 2009.

Gaba, David M. Crisis management in anesthesiology. 2nd edn. New York: Churchill Livingstone, 2009.

Oberoi G, Phillips GD, eds. Anaesthesia and emergency situations: a management guide. Sydney: McGraw-Hill Book Company, 2000.

Data interpretation

Bonner S, Dodds C, eds. Clinical data interpretation in anaesthesia and intensive care. Edinburgh: Churchill Livingstone, 2002.

Hobbs G, Mahajan R. Imaging in anaesthesia and critical care. London: Churchill Livingstone, 2000.

Day surgery anaesthesia

Shapiro FE, ed. Manual of office-based anesthesia procedures. Philadelphia: Wolters Kluwer – Lippincott Williams and Wilkins, 2007.

Smith I, ed. Day care anaesthesia. London: BMJ, 2000.

Steele SM, Nielsen KC, Klein SM, eds. Ambulatory anesthesia and perioperative analgesia. New York: McGraw-Hill, 2005.

White PF, ed. Ambulatory anesthesia and surgery. London: W B Saunders, 1997.

Equipment

Brimacombe JR. Laryngeal mask anaesthesia: principles and practice. 2nd edn. Philadelphia: Saunders, 2005.

Davey A, Ward C S, eds. Ward's anaesthetic equipment. 5th edn. London: W B Saunders, 2005.

Dorsch JA, Dorsch SE. Understanding anesthesia equipment. 5th edn. Philadelphia: Lippincott Williams and Wilkins, 2008.

Russell WJ. Equipment for anaesthesia and intensive care. 2nd edn. Adelaide: W J Russell, 1997.

Sykes MK, Vickers MD, Hull CJ. Principles of measurement and monitoring in anaesthesia and intensive care. 3rd edn. London: Blackwell Scientific Publications, 1991.

Intensive care

Bersten AD, Soni N, eds. Oh's intensive care manual. 6th edn. Edinburgh: Butterworth-Heinemann Elsevier, 2009.

Blackwell N, Foot C, Thomas C. Examination intensive care and anaesthesia: A guide to intensivist and anaesthetist training. Sydney: Churchill Livingstone-Elsevier, 2007.

Hall JB, Schmidt GA, Wood LDH, eds. Principles of critical care. 3rd edn. New York: McGraw-Hill, 2005.

Hillman K, Bishop G. Clinical intensive care and acute medicine. 2nd edn. Melbourne: Cambridge University Press, 2004.

Irwin RS, Rippe JM, eds. Irwin and Rippe's intensive care medicine. Philadelphia: Wolters Kluwer – Lippincott Williams and Wilkins, 2008.

Marino PL. The ICU book. 3rd edn. Philadelphia: Lippincott Williams and Wilkins, 2007.

Neuroanaesthesia

Gupta AK, Gelb AW. Essentials of neuroanesthesia and neurointensive care. Philadelphia, PA: Elsevier Saunders, 2008.

Matta BF, Menon DK, Turner JM, eds. Textbook of neuroanaesthesia and critical care. London: Greenwich Medical Media, 2000.

Newfield P, Cottrell JE, eds. Handbook of neuroanesthesia. 3rd edn. Philadelphia: Lippincott Williams and Wilkins, 1999.

Obstetric anaesthesia

Chestnut DH, ed. Obstetric anesthesia: principles and practice. 3rd edn. Philadelphia: Elsevier Mosby, 2004.

Clyburn P, Collis R, Harries S, Davies S, eds. Obstetric anaesthesia. New York: Oxford University Press, 2008.

Collis RE, Plaat F, Urquhart J, eds. Textbook of obstetric anaesthesia. London: Greenwich Medical Media, 2002.

Gambling DR, Douglas MJ, McKay RSF, eds. Obstetric anesthesia and uncommon disorders. 2nd edn. Cambridge: Cambridge University Press, 2008.

Halpern SH, Douglas MJ, eds. Evidence-based obstetric anesthesia. Massachusetts: Blackwell Publishing, 2005.

Hughes SC, Levinson G, Rosen M, eds. Shnider and Levinson's anesthesia for obstetrics. 4th edn. Philadelphia: Lippincott Williams & Wilkins, 2002.

Paediatric anaesthesia

Black AE, McEwan A. Paediatric and neonatal anaesthesia. Edinburgh: Butterworth Heinemann, 2004.

Cotè CJ, ed. A practice of anesthesia for infants and children. 3rd edn. Philadelphia: WB Saunders, 2001.

Doyle E, ed. Paediatric anaesthesia. Oxford: Oxford University Press, 2007.

Motoyama EK, Davis PJ, eds. Smith's anesthesia for infants and children. 7th edn. Philadelphia: Mosby, 2006.

Steward DJ, Lerman J. Manual of pediatric anesthesia. 5th edn. New York: Churchill Livingstone, 2001.

Pain management

Breivik H, Campbell W, Nicholas MK, eds. Clinical pain management: practice and procedures. 2nd edn. London: Hodder Arnold, 2008.

Coniam S, Mendham J. Principles of pain management for anaesthetists. London: Hodder Arnold, 2006.

Macintyre PE, Schug S. Acute pain management: a practical guide. 3rd edn. Edinburgh: Elsevier Saunders, 2007.

Macintyre PE, Walker SM, Rowbotham DJ, eds. Clinical pain management: acute pain. 2nd edn. London: Hodder Arnold, 2008.

McMahon SB, Koltzenburg M, eds. Wall and Melzack's textbook of pain. 5th edn. New York: Elsevier Churchill Livingstone, 2005.

Sykes N, Bennett MI, Yuan C-S, eds. Clinical pain management: cancer pain. 2nd edn. London: Hodder Arnold, 2008.

Waldman SD. Atlas of common pain syndromes. 2nd edn. Philadelphia: Elsevier Saunders, 2008.

Waldman SD. Atlas of uncommon pain syndromes. 2nd edn. Philadelphia: Elsevier Saunders, 2008.

Wilson PR, Watson PJ, Haythornthwaite JA, Jensen TS, eds. Clinical pain management: chronic pain. London: Hodder Arnold, 2008.

Perioperative medicine

Cashman JN, ed. Preoperative assessment. London: BMJ Books, 2001.

Hines R, Marschall K, eds. Stoelting's anesthesia and co-existing disease. 5th edn. Philadelphia: Churchill Livingstone, 2008.

Sweitzer B, ed. Preoperative assessment and management. 2nd edn. Philadelphia: Lippincott Williams and Wilkins, 2008.

Talley NJ, O'Connor S. Clinical examination: a systematic guide to physical diagnosis. 6th edn. Sydney: Churchill Livingstone Elsevier, 2009.

Talley NJ, O'Connor S. Examination medicine: a guide to physician training. 6th edn. Sydney: Churchill Livingstone Elsevier, 2010.

Principles of anaesthesia practice

Aitkenhead AR, Smith G, Rowbotham DJ, eds. Textbook of anaesthesia. 5th edn. Edinburgh: Churchill Livingstone, 2007.

Barash PG, Cullen BF, Stoelting RK, Cahalan MK, Stock MC, eds. Clinical anesthesia. Philadelphia: Lippincott Williams and Wilkins, 2009.

Davies NJH, Cashman JN, eds. Lee's synopsis of anaesthesia. 13th edn. Oxford: Butterworth-Heinemann, 2005.

Fleisher, Lee A, ed. Evidence-based practice of anesthesiology. 2nd edn. Philadelphia: Elsevier Saunders, 2009.

Jaffe RA, Samuels SI, eds. Anesthesiologist's manual of surgical procedures. 4th edn. Philadelphia: Wolters Kluwer–Lippincott Williams and Wilkins, 2009.

Miller RD, ed. Miller's anesthesia. 7th edn. Philadelphia: Elsevier Churchill Livingstone, 2009.

Morgan GED, Mikhail MS, Murray MJ, eds. Clinical anesthesiology. 4th edn. New York: Lange Medical Books/McGraw-Hill, 2006.

Smith T, Pinnock C, Lin T, eds. Fundamentals of anaesthesia. Cambridge: Cambridge University Press, 2009.

Yao F-S, Malhotra V, Fontes ML, eds. Yao and Artusio's anesthesiology: problem-oriented patient management. 6th edn. Philadelphia: Lippincott Williams and Wilkins, 2008.

Yentis SM, Hirsch NP, Smith GB. Anaesthesia and intensive care A–Z: an encyclopaedia of principles and practice. 4th edn. Edinburgh: Churchill Livingstone, 2009.

Regional anaesthesia

Barrett J, Harmon D, Loughnane F, Finucane BT, Shorten G. Peripheral nerve blocks and peri-operative pain relief. Edinburgh: Saunders, 2004.

Brown DL. Atlas of regional anesthesia. 3rd edn. Philadelphia: Elsevier Saunders, 2006.

Chelly JE, ed. Peripheral nerve blocks: a color atlas. 3rd edn. Philadelphia: Lippincott Williams and Wilkins, 2009.

Cousins MJ, Carr DB, Horlocker TT, Bridenbaugh PO, eds. Cousins and Bridenbaugh's neural blockade in clinical anesthesia and pain medicine. 4th edn. Philadelphia: Wolters Kluwer – Lippincott Williams and Wilkins, 2009.

Hadzic A, ed. Textbook of regional anesthesia and acute pain management. New York: McGraw-Hill Medical, 2007.

Marhofer P. Ultrasound guidance for nerve blocks: principles and practical implementation. Oxford: Oxford University Press, 2008.

Mulroy MF. Regional anesthesia: an illustrated procedural guide. 3rd edn. Philadelphia: Lippincott Williams and Wilkins, 2002.

Mulroy MF, Bernards CM, McDonald SB, Salinas FV, eds. A practical guide to regional anesthesia. 4th edn. Baltimore: Lippincott Williams and Wilkins, 2009.

Wildsmith JAW, ed. Principles and practice of regional anesthesia. 3rd edn. London: Churchill Livingstone, 2003.

Statistics and research

Dawson B, Trapp RG. Basic and clinical biostatistics. 4th edn. New York: Lange Medical Books – McGraw-Hill, 2004.

Myles PS, Gin T. Statistical methods for anaesthesia and intensive care. Sydney: Butterworth Heinemann, 2000.

Zbinden AM, Thomson D, eds. Conducting research in anaesthesia and intensive care medicine. Oxford: Butterworth Heinemann, 2001.

Journals

It is important for candidates to conduct an appraisal of contemporary anaesthetic research. Review articles are also published regularly in the major journals, and serve as a useful tool for reviewing important topics. The journals and periodicals form a good base on which to draw:

- *Acta Anaesthesiologica Scandinavica*
- *Anaesthesia*
- *Anaesthesia and Intensive Care*
- *Anesthesia and Analgesia*
- *Anesthesiology*
- *Anesthesiology Clinics of North America*
- *Australasian Anaesthesia* (published every second year – the 'blue book', now available online)
- *British Journal of Anaesthesia*
- *Canadian Journal of Anaesthesia*
- *Continuing Education in Anaesthesia, Critical Care and Pain* (published by the *British Journal of Anaesthesia*)
- *Current Opinion in Anesthesiology*
- *The Lancet*
- *New England Journal of Medicine*
- *Paediatric Anaesthesia*
- *Regional Anaesthesia and Pain Medicine*

A summary of many recent useful reference and review articles is provided in Chapter 7.

Resuscitation guidelines

Crisis management forms an integral part of the working knowledge of the anaesthetist, and a very high standard of expertise in this area is expected of candidates in the final examination. Candidates should have a comprehensive knowledge of currently accepted standards in first aid and resuscitation.

The Australian Resuscitation Council publishes its guidelines as an online resource, available at www.resus.org.au. These guidelines are regularly updated (the last major overhaul was in 2006, but individual components may be updated more frequently). They encompass principles of basic life support, such as management of the unconscious victim, airway, breathing and circulation (including cardiopulmonary resuscitation algorithms), other specific first aid emergencies (such as envenomation, burns and shock), and detailed guidelines on advanced life support techniques for adults, children and neonates.

The New Zealand Resuscitation Council guidelines, which are available at www.nzrc.org.nz, are somewhat less comprehensive and contain some minor differences from their Australian counterparts. Algorithms are presented for adult and child resuscitation, and the use of automatic defibrillators is discussed. Examiners are aware of minor regional differences in recommended resuscitation pathways, and are able to take these into account where relevant.

Courses

Several courses are offered throughout Australia and New Zealand to help candidates prepare for the final examination.

Long courses usually consist of interactive lectures on broad topics related to the examination and are held once a week or once a fortnight for several hours. These courses usually run all year round and serve as a good companion to general study for the examination. While they can help candidates focus their attention on key areas, most benefit will be obtained from them if you are already familiar with the material when attending the lecture. Attendance at these courses is often limited by candidates' geographical location.

Short courses are usually run over one or two weeks and are intensely exam focused, often including practice examinations, vivas and even medical cases. Topics are presented in a more interactive format than in the long courses, and tend to concentrate on areas relevant to the examination. Presenters on these courses are often final examiners. Numbers for many short courses are strictly limited, and preference is often given to candidates from the local area and those who are definitely sitting the next examination, so it is important to carefully check the opening and closing dates for applications. When choosing a course it is important to talk to colleagues who have recently attended them to gain an appreciation of the relative strengths and weaknesses different courses may have. Ideally, you should have most of the knowledge you need before attending the course. What you are aiming to achieve is a refinement of this knowledge and a honing of your examination techniques. The opportunity to see where you are in relation to other candidates is also useful.

Trial vivas are held in several centres and offer the opportunity for practice in the simulated stress of the examination, free of charge. They usually provide an opportunity for trainees who are not yet ready to take the exam to observe others in action.

The following courses are currently offered in Australia and New Zealand. Please contact the co-ordinators of these courses or regional committees for more details.

NSW
Contact: nswcourses@anzca.edu.au

Part II refresher course	February	Royal Prince Alfred Hospital, Sydney
ANZCA Part II short course	June	Westmead Hospital, Sydney

NZ
Contact: training@anzca.org.nz

Oral examination course	February/July	Wellington
Part II two-week short course	June–July	Auckland

QLD
Contact: qldcourses@anzca.edu.au

Part II one-week short course	February/July	Brisbane
Final examination lecture program	One night/month (February, May, August, November)	Brisbane

SA / NT
Contact: sa@anzca.edu.au

Part II preparation lecture course	February–November (Fridays 13.30–17.00)	Various hospitals

VIC
Contact: viccourses@anzca.edu.au

Final full-time one-week course	February/July	ANZCA House
Final medical refresher	February/July (Four consecutive Saturday mornings)	Metro hospitals
Final anatomy one-day course	May/October	ANZCA House

WA

Contact: wa@anzca.edu.au

Part II tutorials	All year (18.30 Tuesday or Wednesday)	Royal Perth/Sir Charles Gairdner Hospitals

Informal tutorials on areas of interest are also provided by anaesthetists at many hospitals. Details of these should be available from supervisors of training at the respective hospitals.

Preparation strategies

Philosophy

The final examination in anaesthesia is daunting for most candidates. This is a test of your ability to demonstrate your knowledge and apply it to being a safe consultant. A very high standard is required to achieve a passing grade.

It must be stressed that the time and effort taken in preparing for the final examination is really an investment in becoming a better anaesthetist. Candidates who study purely with the aim of achieving a passing grade in the exam sometimes lose sight of this fact, and limit their acquisition of knowledge to a superficial coverage of many topics. The best performance in the examination on any particular topic is achieved by those candidates who have read about a subject, thought about it critically, and ideally had exposure to the situation in clinical practice.

While you will be challenged on a wide variety of subspecialty areas the examiners are not looking to see if you are an authority on every topic, but that you have been given an adequate exposure to these areas during your training and have a grasp of important concepts. If you can draw on your previous experiences when answering a question, so much the better. It is likely, though, that you will encounter scenarios you have never seen in real life. Through your appraisal of texts and current literature, and from a sound grasp of first principles, you should be able to construct a sensible approach to the management of such cases.

The tone you must adopt in the examination (both written and clinical) is one of the authority of a specialist, without appearing arrogant. To an outside observer, the viva examination should appear to be a considered discussion between colleagues. The persona of the timid trainee will not win you many points in the clinical exam. The examiners are able to assess your ability to handle internal stress and external pressure, which may be extrapolated (perhaps unfairly) to mirror your performance as an anaesthetist.

Timing

The college recommends that you begin preparation for the final examination as soon as you complete the primary examination. It is wise to peruse past examiners' reports and the college trainee support kit to gain an appreciation of the scope of the exam, and then begin collating resources. Work out when it is optimal for you to sit the exam. The beginning of the second advanced vocational training year is favoured by many candidates as it offers them a balance between plenty of preparation time and the 'luxury' of further attempts should they be unsuccessful, without adding to their total training time. It may be helpful to plan your study around the nearest long course the year before the exam. Approximately one year of intensive study seems to be a good average to obtain a satisfactory standard, but this will vary from trainee to trainee. If you decide to work through the entire multiple choice question bank on your own, you will need approximately 15 months. This is one area where working in a study group will save you considerable time.

Most candidates focus on the written components of the examination (especially the multiple choice questions) in the lead-up to the exam, then work on their viva technique in the six weeks before the clinical exam. This approach is usually successful. One advantage of subjecting yourself to viva scenarios before the written examination is that it may force you to think in a more logical, sequential and coherent manner, which can be of some benefit for structuring answers in the short answer section of the examination. Do not leave it too late to practise medical viva cases, as smooth patient evaluation and presentation techniques are of paramount importance for negotiating this section of the exam. The recent restructuring of the exam chronology means that these techniques will be on show just one day after the written exam.

Study groups

How you study for the examination is an intensely personal decision, and there is no right or wrong approach. Some candidates are more efficient at digesting a large amount of material by themselves, while others work better in groups where some of the workload can be divided. The group approach has its advantages when you are battling through thousands of multiple choice questions, as previously mentioned.

The study group may be an effective forum for sharing information and ideas. There is much to be learnt from others, and the social and emotional support that you can gain from your colleagues can be invaluable in helping you cope with the stress of exam preparation. When a workload is shared there may be additional motivation to study effectively, so as not to let the group down. The most successful study groups will give each participant an active role.

There may be a limit to the number your group can accommodate, as it depends on many factors (e.g. how many from your region are sitting the exam or who is interested). Even a study pair may be of benefit.

If working in a study group beware of time inefficiency and distractions. Your group must be focused on the goal and how to achieve it, so some planning is essential. How often you meet and for how long are important. Divide up the work to be covered so it is all handled efficiently. Decide on what is important for the group to cover and what can be done alone. Some groups simply focus on one aspect of the exam, such as multiple choice questions or literature searching, with individuals of the group completing the remainder of their study alone.

The group must be like-minded in their philosophy with the aim of helping everyone. Highly competitive members will not help you if their aim is to outperform other members of the group. Be aware that everyone has their own preferences and rate of learning. Work out ways to handle arguments, discussions and delays. It is important for the group to solve group dynamic problems early on.

Looking after yourself

Adjusting your personal life around the examination can be difficult. How you and your family cope with this stress can play a large part in your chances of success at the examination and how the rest of your life continues afterwards.

Your immediate family may already have an idea of what to expect if they experienced your efforts at the primary examination. Try and explain the scope of what is involved. Partners play an important role by providing social support and helping with emotional problems. You must sacrifice much of your time and attention to study, which is often a source of great stress to your significant other (who is also making great sacrifices to give you the time to study). Preparation for the final exam is often emotionally more difficult for the partner who is not sitting it. Plan some time every week to spend with other family members.

All of us cope with stress in a different way. Meditation, yoga or exercise may be all that you need to maintain a relaxed and balanced life. Psychologists and counselling may help if you are not coping so well. Avoid relying on cigarettes, alcohol and other recreational pharmacology as a means of coping. Eat sensibly and healthily, and exercise a few times a week. There is no point flogging your mind with hours of study a day if your body collapses and is unable to sustain the effort.

The time you spend at work can be used to your advantage in preparing for the examination. Question everything you do. When supervised, ask your consultants to question you on various topics and challenge you on the management of patients on the operating list. Use your preoperative assessments or pre-admission clinics as practice for the medical vivas. If possible, present your findings to a colleague (time restraints of a busy clinic may not always permit this). Ask your colleagues to be on the lookout for interesting medical cases and enlist the help of a friendly intensivist or physician colleague for short case practice. If supervising a junior trainee, use the teaching time as a presentation or dissertation of important information (as you might in the exam).

In summary, you must negotiate the difficult but important apportioning of your time among work, study, recreation and family. Talking to your colleagues, supervisor of training or someone within the college may be useful in helping you plan different strategies for dealing with exam preparation.

Coping with failure

Failure at the final examination is a difficult thing to cope with, but is a concept that confronts every candidate. Because of the breadth of the testing process for the final exam, candidates who have devoted the appropriate amount of time to study and who are well prepared through practice will almost always be successful. It is possible to have a difficult viva early in the clinical exam, which can throw your performance for the rest of the day. In addition, candidates with great knowledge sometimes simply freeze in the stress of the situation and do not do themselves justice by their performance. Concurrent illness, difficulties with English and external life stresses may also thwart otherwise well-prepared candidates.

Overwhelming sadness, anger and a depressed mood are common among those who have not passed. There is often a feeling of having let oneself and one's family down when a great deal has already been sacrificed. The financial loss is significant, especially for those candidates who have travelled from interstate and overseas. There is also the worry of what colleagues and consultants may say at work, and a feeling of inferiority for not having made the grade. Colleagues who have passed the exam may not be able to relate well to you – they want to celebrate themselves, but at the same time do not want to be seen to be celebrating your misery. Finally, there is still a mountain to climb to pass the exam next time.

Overseas trained specialists may face additional pressures and problems. Employment positions and work visas often hinge on the outcome of the examination. The scope and focus of the final examination may be considerably different from the specialist examinations of their home country, and a failure to appreciate this may hamper their chances of passing on the first attempt.

Fortunately, most candidates who fail the exam pass easily on their next sitting. The college is kind enough to provide a written breakdown of marks, and now offers a feedback interview to assist candidates in preparing for future exams. The majority of people who fail do so at the written exam, and supervisors of training may be able to help with strategies and extra tutorials to augment knowledge, answer structure and overall performance in this area.

Remember that failing the final exam is not a unique experience, and many fine anaesthetists have transiently stumbled at this hurdle. Using the experience gained during the first attempt should help candidates prepare for the subsequent one. Persistence is the key, and if a candidate's desire to complete the FANZCA program is strong enough, the final examination is unlikely to be unconquered for long.

Chapter 3

The written examination

Common sense is not so common.
VOLTAIRE

Overview

More so than the clinical sections of the examination, the two written components test not only the candidate's knowledge, but their ability to effectively manage time. Candidates are given two and a half hours to complete each of the exam papers, which places the responsibility for time management squarely on the shoulders of the candidate, unlike the rapid-fire 18- or 15-minute medical and anaesthesia vivas, each of which passes by in a blur. The keys to success in the written section are discipline and practice. Examination time must be ruthlessly allocated, so that an equal amount is given to each question, especially in the short answer section.

Each written paper is worth 20% of the final examination mark. Candidates are not obliged to pass either to pass the exam as a whole, but if they fail both, as well as the medical vivas, they will not be invited to sit the anaesthesia viva component. Performing poorly in both written sections also puts enormous pressure on a candidate for the remaining sections of the examination.

The multiple choice questions test a broad range of topics and their minutiae, and are useful administrative tools for distinguishing between very good and very poor candidates. As a significant number of questions are repeated between exams, they also offer candidates the opportunity to collect some 'free' marks, if their revision of past papers has been well-organised and comprehensive.

The short answer questions are a test not only of knowledge but of organisation and clear thinking. Candidates who present their answers with a logical sequence, usefully categorised or in tabular form may score more marks than someone who has exactly the same information recorded as a random flight of ideas on the page.

Performance strategies

Double-check the date, time and venue of the exam the week before. Resist the urge to study the day before the examination (which is usually on a Friday). If possible, you should be well rested and relaxed, so get as much sleep the night before as your adrenal glands will allow. If you have travelled from a peripheral centre to sit the exam, try to arrive early the day before. Don't skimp on the cost of accommodation as you should aim for as peaceful a night's rest as possible.

In the past, candidates have set two alarm clocks to avoid the embarrassment and catastrophic consequences of sleeping in.

Allow yourself plenty of time for breakfast and the journey to the exam destination, including catching a taxi or finding a car park (if your venue does not provide ample parking). The first written paper is normally due to start at the end of peak-hour traffic. Make sure you have your candidate number and some form of photo identification (preferably a driver's licence or passport) with you. Take a selection of pens, pencils (2B), a pencil sharpener, a new eraser, a ruler and a digital watch with a stopwatch function. The examination venue will provide you with pencils and an eraser for the exam if you don't have your own. Leave all of your textbooks, multiple choice question bank and other study notes at home.

Try and arrive at the venue with at least half an hour to spare. Take a few quiet moments just before you enter the exam to think positive thoughts and clear your head. It is amazing how quickly your nerves and anxiety will dissipate once the exam begins (usually after you recognise a couple of repeat multiple choice questions on the first page).

Before you commence the exam you must sign on with the invigilators, who will check your identification and examination number against the photographic college record. You will be directed to your seat, which is marked with your examination number.

Multiple choice questions (MCQ)

Make sure that you correctly enter your name and examination number on the answer sheet. This is especially important because all of the answer sheets are marked by computer. In the event that an answer sheet contains major irregularities (e.g. no responses are registered by the computer or there are lengthy sequences of consecutive incorrect responses), it may be manually checked. Once you have filled in the required information you will be given instructions on the timing of the examination. When the perusal time starts, start the timer on your digital watch so you can keep an eye on this as you work (the clock in the room is not always easily visible to all candidates).

Time management is critical, as there is one minute per multiple choice question. In the perusal time candidates are given 10 minutes head-start on the race with the clock, during which time notes may be made on the examination paper (but *not* on the answer sheet).

Because of the marking system used by the examiners, it is in your best interests to attempt every question. Marks are not deducted for mistakes. For questions you do not know the answer to, eliminate whatever alternatives you can and then take a guess. Acknowledge this is a guess by resisting the temptation to change the answer later, unless there is a good reason to do so. Read every question carefully, and consider underlining or highlighting words such as 'except', 'usually', 'maybe' and 'never', and phrases that contain double negatives.

It is probably wise to attempt all questions in order. Most candidates will transcribe the answers from those questions completed in the perusal time onto the answer sheet when time proper commences, and then continue answering questions directly onto the answer sheet. An alternative approach is to continue to answer all the questions by annotating the question paper, then transcribe all 150 answers onto the answer sheet at the end. The advantage of this latter approach is that you are less likely to commit a sequence error if you consciously transcribe and check in blocks of 5 or

10 questions. Also, if there is a question that you are unsure of you can indicate this with a big question mark and move on (rather than leaving a single answer line unfilled and forgetting to come back to it), taking your best guess at it when you return to it in the transcription process. The disadvantage of this approach is that if time runs short you may be left with a larger chunk of unanswered questions at the end of your answer sheet.

Follow the instructions on the answer sheet carefully. Answers are recorded by completely shading the appropriate area on the answer paper in pencil. The papers are marked by computer, so be careful when filling in the small ovals, especially when changing an answer (be sure to completely erase your previous response; if the computer detects two responses it will be marked as wrong). Check the question and answer numbers every five questions or so to avoid a sequence error. It takes a very long time to change half the answers simply because one was left out somewhere along the way.

Hand in all papers at the end of the exam. All of the multiple-choice question papers are coded with your examination number and if you remove one from the examination room you will automatically fail.

You will have a couple of free hours between the two written exams. Try and avoid a post-mortem dissection of the MCQ exam with colleagues, as this achieves nothing.

Go for a walk in the vicinity of the venue to clear your head, and try to eat a light lunch. Return to the examination venue with plenty of time to spare. Take a few quiet moments just before you enter the exam to think positive thoughts and clear your head (again).

Short answer questions (SAQ)

Take time before you commence the short answer paper to ensure your candidate number and the correct question number is written on the front page of each answer book (15 in all).

For the short answer paper, time management cannot be overemphasised. You must ruthlessly adhere to the 10-minute time limit per question as it is unlikely the extra marks you score in going overtime in one question will compensate for those lost through lack of time in another. Even the outline of an answer containing a few key points may score 1 or 2 marks; the same time spent enhancing an already acceptable answer may not actually improve its score.

A recurring comment in examiners' reports is the failure of candidates to answer what is asked. An erudite dissertation on a topic scores no points if it does not directly answer the question posed. Read each question carefully, then read it again. Underline the key points of a question on the question paper, and jot down a quick plan or structure for your answer. Be especially aware of instructions such as *compare, contrast, justify, describe* and *list*, and make sure your answer adequately complies with such requests. Keep an open mind and consider the broadest possible approach to each question. Construct your answers logically. Where possible, list points under headings and categories. This is more efficient than freehand prose and immediately simplifies the examiners' task of awarding you marks. A well-defined structure that answers all aspects of the question is the key to gaining marks.

Do not write things that will irritate the examiners. They expect a professional response to the problem posed, commensurate with the mature thinking of a consultant anaesthetist. Unwarranted personal opinions, wisecracks, offensive language and sarcasm are not appropriate; they will also be recorded permanently and cannot be withdrawn. Do not draw cartoons or smiley faces in the answer books. Avoid the use of abbreviations that may be open to interpretation (alternatively, define each abbreviation the first time it is used in the text of your answer). Examiners have specifically commented on the futility of using the term 'etc.' in an answer, and that the term 'consider' in response to a question on emergency management does not inspire confidence.

Write as neatly as possible. The examiners go to extraordinary lengths to decipher poor handwriting, but even they have limits. The answer books provided by the college have very widely spaced lines, which may encourage more legible writing. It may consequently be useful for you to practise using only every third line of standard-ruled paper. Do not worry if you fill an answer book – you will be provided with another (but remember to fill in your details on the front). Advise the invigilators at the end of the exam that you have used two books for one question and they will staple them together.

It is very important to only answer one question per answer book. Do not cross-reference your answers as they will be marked by different examiners.

It is generally only appropriate to quote articles from the literature if you can cite them perfectly (a difficult feat to achieve). The majority of short answer questions do not require such supporting information. However, there have been some questions in recent years that have asked for knowledge of landmark research to justify a response or point of view.

At the end of the exam be sure your candidate number is on every answer book and that they are all are returned to the invigilators. There are several recent tales of candidates who have discovered one of the answer books (usually with their best answer) still among their possessions when they have arrived home from the exam. The invigilators now check to see if all books have been returned, but ultimately the responsibility rests with the candidate. You are allowed to remove the short answer question paper from the examination room.

Go home and get some rest. You have another big day tomorrow.

Written examination topics

The following section lists the short answer questions from the most recent five years (2005–09). These have been sorted into relevant topic headings. Each question is followed by the sitting number (1 or 2) and year of origin.

Airway management
- How do you assess a patient at the bedside with regard to difficulty of intubation? How accurate is such an assessment? (1/07)
- Describe your immediate assessment and management of the airway in a patient with smoke inhalation injury. (1/06)
- What is the role of a laryngeal mask airway in a failed intubation for laparotomy? (2/05)

Ambulatory anaesthesia
- A fit 18-year-old is to have wisdom teeth removed as a day-stay patient. Describe and justify features of your anaesthetic technique that may help prevent common postoperative problems you would anticipate in this patient. (2/07)

- Discuss the role of non-steroidal anti-inflammatory agents for postoperative analgesia in adult day-stay patients. (1/06)
- How would you manage the discovery of a small pneumothorax in a 35-year-old female following removal of a breast lump under local anaesthesia in a day surgery facility? (2/05)

Anaesthetic equipment

- Describe the differences between biphasic and monophasic manual external cardiac defibrillators. What is the 'synchronize' button for and when would you use it? List the potential hazards of defibrillation. (2/09)
- Define decontamination, disinfection and sterilisation. Outline measures to reduce the risk of transmission of infection to a patient's respiratory tract from anaesthetic equipment. (1/09)
- What are essential safety requirements for delivery of gases from anaesthetic machines and breathing circuits? (1/09)
- Outline operating principles and safety features of a modern variable bypass vaporiser. (2/08)
- Outline storage and delivery of oxygen to theatre. Include safety features of the system. (1/08)
- Explain the features of the electrical power supply to operating theatres that protect patients from macroshock. (2/07)
- Describe the technique of chest tube insertion and the features of a pleural drainage system to treat a large haemo/pneumothorax after attempted left subclavian dialysis access. (2/07)
- How does soda lime work? List the hazards associated with its use. (1/07)
- 'The T-piece is obsolete in modern anaesthesia practice.' Discuss. (1/07)
- Draw a circle breathing system and give reasons for the location of the components. (1/05)

Applied anatomy

- Identify labelled cardiac and vascular structures on a normal chest X-ray. Describe the arterial blood supply and venous drainage of the myocardium. (2/09)
- Draw a cross-section of the arm at the level of the axilla showing anatomy relevant to brachial plexus blockade. List advantages and disadvantages of block at this level versus supraclavicular block. (1/09)
- Draw bronchial anatomy to the level of lobar bronchi and describe use of fibre-optic bronchoscopy to position a right-sided double lumen tube. (1/09)
- Describe the innervation of the lower anterior abdominal wall. Describe a technique of peripheral nerve block to analgese a low transverse abdominal incision. (2/08)
- Why is the radial artery a common site for arterial cannulation? What complications may occur and how may they be minimised? (1/08)
- Describe brachial plexus anatomy relevant to performing interscalene block under ultrasound guidance. Draw real or sono-anatomy you would expect in transverse view of the plexus at the point of needle insertion. (1/08)
- Describe the blood supply to the spinal cord. Explain the determinants of spinal cord perfusion. (2/07)
- Describe the relevant anatomy of the popliteal fossa and a technique of neural blockade in the region for surgery on the foot and ankle. (2/07)

- Describe the relevant anatomy and technique for field block for inguinal hernia repair. (1/07)
- Describe the anatomy of the orbit relevant to a peribulbar eye block. (1/06)
- Describe the anatomy of the trigeminal nerve relevant to local anaesthesia for dental extraction. (2/05)
- Describe the symptoms and signs of commonly seen perioperative nerve injuries in the upper limb. List causes and possible strategies for prevention. (2/05)
- Outline the anatomy of the right internal jugular vein as it is relevant to your preferred method of percutaneous cannulation. (1/05)

Applied physiology and pharmacology

- Outline the factors that determine oxygen delivery to the tissues. How might you increase tissue oxygen delivery in an anaesthetised patient? How does a hyperbaric chamber influence tissue oxygen delivery? (2/09)
- Describe the characteristics of remifentanil with respect to its use in an infusion. What are the advantages and disadvantages of using effect site calculations to guide remifentanil infusions? (2/09)
- Describe the mechanism and duration of action of clopidogrel. (2/09)
- Describe the physiological effects of pneumoperitoneum with carbon dioxide for laparoscopic surgery. (1/09)
- Discuss the pros and cons of intrathecal morphine for postoperative analgesia for total knee replacement surgery. (1/08)
- Discuss the statement: 'It is no longer justifiable to use aprotinin during cardiac surgical procedures'. (2/07)
- 'Nitrous oxide should not be used routinely as a component of general anaesthesia'. Discuss. (2/06)
- Discuss the role of ketamine in current anaesthesia practice. (2/06)
- What is the physiological basis of preoxygenation? Describe your method of preoxygenation and how you assess its adequacy. (1/06)
- Discuss the role of desflurane in current anaesthesia practice. (1/06)
- How does anaesthesia alter temperature homeostasis? (2/05)
- The hospital pharmacist notifies you as Director of Anaesthesia that thiopentone is to be withdrawn from the hospital due to minimal usage. Outline and justify your response. (2/05)
- List the physiological effects of electroconvulsive therapy and how they may be modified. (2/05)
- What significant side-effects are associated with the use of anti-emetic agents? (1/05)

Crisis management

- An arterial blood gas, showing severe mixed respiratory and metabolic acidoses, is obtained, after several minutes of CPR, from a 70-year-old patient who is in cardiac arrest in recovery after fixation of a femoral fracture. Describe the aetiology and pathogenesis of the abnormalities shown. (2/09)
- A 49-year-old in the recovery room is agitated and complaining of difficulty breathing following abdominal hysterectomy. List a differential diagnosis. How would you determine if this was due to residual neuromuscular blockade? What is the role of sugammadex in this situation? (2/09)

- Outline the management of evolving malignant hyperthermia (scenario given of rising end-tidal carbon dioxide, worsening sinus tachycardia with ventricular ectopy and mixed metabolic and respiratory acidosis). (1/09)
- Discuss the features and the clinical management of amniotic fluid embolism. (1/09)
- Describe the management of respiratory distress in a total thyroidectomy patient in the recovery room. (1/09)
- What would lead you to suspect venous gas embolism during surgery? Outline principles of management. (2/08)
- A 14-year-old boy presents obtunded and hypotensive with a rash suggestive of meningococcal sepsis. Describe your resuscitation. (2/08)
- Describe the features and management of fat embolism syndrome. (1/08)
- A 38-year-old woman is found obtunded 30 hours after abdominal hysterectomy. Describe how severe hyponatraemia and hypoosmolality may have arisen and how you would correct such abnormalities. (1/08)
- A patient is brought to hospital rescued from a swimming pool, followed by CPR from ambulance officers. Describe how basic life support should be provided in the emergency department. The patient has no pulse and the ECG shows ventricular fibrillation. Outline the advanced life support algorithm you would now follow. (1/07)
- Discuss assessment and management of a patient who becomes restless 70 minutes into transurethral prostate resection under spinal anaesthesia, having received 2 mg midazolam at start of the case. (1/06)
- Describe the clinical features and management of bupivacaine toxicity. (1/06)
- How would you diagnose a clinically significant latex allergy occurring intraoperatively? (2/05)
- List the possible causes of failure to emerge from general anaesthesia and describe how you would differentiate them. (1/05)

Intensive care topics

- Explain the problems associated with initiating ventilatory support in a patient with acute severe asthma and describe how you would overcome them. (2/07)
- What are the principles of ventilatory management of patients with acute respiratory distress syndrome? (1/07)
- Discuss the usefulness of the continuous measurement of mixed venous oxygen saturation in the intensive care patient. (1/07)
- Outline the steps necessary to diagnose brain death in a patient comatose following a subarachnoid haemorrhage. (1/07)

Monitoring

- List the patterns of peripheral nerve stimulation used to monitor non-depolarising blockade and describe how each is used in clinical practice. (1/07)
- Describe how the ECG should be used to monitor for intraoperative myocardial ischaemia in a patient with ischaemic heart disease. (1/07)
- Preoperative ECG of 56-year-old diabetic illustrated (showing tri-fascicular block). Intraoperative ECG illustrated (showing complete A–V dissociation). Analyse and describe the ECGs. Outline your management of the latter situation. (1/07)

- List the risks associated with the placement of a central venous catheter. Discuss ways in which these risks may be modified. (2/06)
- Compare the use of a pulmonary artery catheter and transoesophageal echocardiography in evaluating cardiac function intraoperatively. (1/05)

Neuroanaesthesia

- Describe issues and their management for middle cerebral artery clipping following sub-arachnoid haemorrhage. (1/09)
- Discuss the management of cerebral vasospasm following coiling of a cerebral aneurysm. (2/08)
- Discuss the perioperative use of nimodipine for a patient undergoing clipping of a cerebral aneurysm. (1/05)

Obstetric anaesthesia

- A 32-week pregnant 150 kg patient has gestational diabetes. She is hoping to have a normal vaginal delivery at term. What are the issues you would discuss with her during the pre-admission appointment? What would you recommend for her management when she goes into labour? (2/09)
- Outline the management of a patient presenting at 38 weeks gestation with features of severe pre-eclampsia. (2/08)
- Describe your pre- and intra-operative management plan for caesarean section for a woman with anterior placenta praevia and a history of two prior caesarean sections. (1/08)
- Describe and justify your choice of drugs and mode of administration of epidural analgesia for a 3 cm dilated primigravida. (2/07)
- You cause inadvertant dural puncture with Tuohy needle performing epidural anaesthesia for first stage primigravida. Describe and justify your management of this complication. (2/06)

Paediatric and neonatal anaesthesia

- You are asked to give a practical tutorial on paediatric airway management to emergency department registrars at a large hospital. What are the important aspects of paediatric airway management that you would present to them? (2/09)
- What is the APGAR score of a baby one minute old who is apnoeic, grey/blue all over, floppy and unresponsive to stimulation with a pulse of 60/min? Describe your resuscitation. (1/08)
- A three-year-old scheduled for dental extractions is found to have a systolic murmur on the day of surgery. Describe how you would evaluate its significance and how the evaluation would affect your decision to proceed or not with surgery. (1/08)
- Describe how the abnormal blood chemistry results (given) arise in pyloric stenosis in infants. Describe an appropriate fluid regimen, and list laboratory criteria by which you would consider a child sufficiently resuscitated for surgery. (2/07)
- Describe the assessment of a two-year-old child with lower body immersion burns, and management of pain and fluid requirements in first two hours following injury. (1/07)
- Discuss in detail the technique of rapid sequence induction with cricoid pressure in a child. Include the reasons for your choice of relaxant. (2/06)

- What are the indications for tracheal intubation in a three-year-old who presents with croup? Describe your technique for intubation. (2/05)

Pain management

- Classify drugs used in pain management according to their safety for use in a 10-week pregnant patient with a closed tibial shaft fracture. What options are available for perioperative pain management of this patient? Justify what you would choose. (2/09)
- A young healthy male has persistent pain 12 weeks after a leg fracture, and is currently taking slow- and immediate-release oxycodone. Discuss the advantages and disadvantages of switching to methadone in this situation and how this may be safely achieved. (1/09)
- List the risk factors for development of chronic pain following a surgical procedure. Outline possible mechanisms for the progression of acute to chronic pain. (2/08)
- Evaluate the role of gabapentin in acute and chronic post-surgical pain management. (1/08)
- Describe the features and management of phantom limb pain. (2/06)
- Discuss the requirements for, and limitations of, the use of patient-controlled analgesia as a technique. (1/05)

Perioperative medicine

- A patient has smoked 20 cigarettes a day for over 25 years. What are the expected physiological changes that would occur in the first three months following cessation of smoking, including a time frame for these changes? What are the clinical benefits, with regard to anaesthesia, of smoking cessation in this patient? (2/09)
- What are the indications for prophylaxis against perioperative bacterial endocarditis? Justify your choice of antibiotics. (2/09)
- List the advantages and disadvantages of tight perioperative glycaemic control on a diabetic patient who is on insulin. How would you manage the glycaemic control of such a patient having a minor procedure under general anaesthesia? (2/09)
- What are the major perioperative considerations for a 70-year-old requiring urgent laparotomy following trauma. She had bare metal coronary stents inserted two months ago and is on clopidogrel. (2/09)
- Discuss issues relevant to the perioperative management of a patient with Parkinson's disease. (1/09)
- Evaluate the usefulness of initiating beta-blocker therapy to prevent myocardial ischaemia in a 65-year-old for surgery for peripheral vascular disease in four days' time. (1/09)
- List and evaluate strategies to prevent perioperative thromboembolism for a patient having radical prostatectomy. (2/08)
- Outline implications of severe spastic cerebral palsy for anaesthesia for major orthopaedic surgery. (2/08)
- What symptoms and signs suggest the presence of sleep apnoea? How does the presence of sleep apnoea alter your anaesthetic plan? (2/08)
- A patient with biventricular failure and an automated implanted cardiac defibrillator presents for elective surgery. Describe how the presence of the device influences your perioperative management. (1/08)

- What are the hazards of laser surgery for a vocal cord papilloma, and how can they be minimised? (1/08)
- Outline the issues in preoperative assessment specific to a patient with acromegaly presenting for transsphenoidal hypophysectomy. (1/08)
- List the problems associated with beach chair position for shoulder surgery and how they may be minimised. (2/07)
- Draw flow-volume loops associated with fixed upper airway obstruction, variable extrathoracic obstruction and variable intrathoracic obstruction, and explain briefly the physiological reasons for the shape of these loops. (2/07)
- Describe the preoperative respiratory evaluation to determine capacity to undergo pneumonectomy for carcinoma in a 65-year-old man with 40-pack-year history of smoking. (1/07)
- Describe methods to optimise the perfusion of a microvascularly implanted forearm in the postoperative period. (1/07)
- Discuss risks and benefits of intermittent positive pressure ventilation through a Proseal® laryngeal mask for laparoscopic cholecystectomy. (2/06)
- List and explain the typical electrolyte abnormalities of chronic renal failure. (2/06)
- Critically evaluate the use of beta blockers in the perioperative period to prevent myocardial infarction. (2/06)
- Discuss the usefulness of the ASA grading as a measure of perioperative risk. (2/06)
- List predisposing factors for aspiration of gastric contents and measures you would take to prevent the complication. (1/06)
- Describe perioperative management of blood sugar for a non-insulin dependent diabetic patient undergoing total abdominal hysterectomy. (1/06)
- Discuss pre- and postoperative management of a patient taking corticosteroid and pyridostigmine for myasthenia gravis. (1/06)
- Discuss relevant factors in your pre-anaesthetic assessment of a patient scheduled to undergo total hip replacement who has a permanent pacemaker. (1/06)
- List the causes of acute atrial fibrillation in the perioperative period. Describe your management if it occurs in recovery in a patient who has had a total hip replacement. (1/06)
- What are the signs, symptoms and anaesthetic implications of autonomic neuropathy associated with diabetes? (2/05)
- Critically evaluate the role of cardioversion in the management of intraoperative arrhythmias. (2/05)
- How would you assess the severity of cardiac failure in a 75-year-old man presenting for joint replacement surgery? (2/05)
- Discuss ways in which the risk of deep venous thrombosis can be minimised in adult patients having intra-abdominal surgery. (1/05)
- What are the problems with the prone position for surgery? (1/05)
- How would you assess a patient's thyroid function preoperatively at the bedside? (1/05)

Regional anaesthesia

- Describe a technique of peribulbar block for cataract surgery. Describe how you would minimise complications of this block. (2/08)

- Outline guidelines to reduce both incidence and morbidity of epidural space infections as a complication of epidural analgesia. (2/07)
- Describe your technique for continuous paravertebral block in a patient with fractured 5th–10th left ribs, including possible complications and relevant anatomy. (2/06)
- Describe and justify a strategy for the use of low molecular weight heparin in a patient undergoing knee replacement surgery with an epidural block. (2/06)
- Discuss the management options for an epidural abscess. (1/05)

Remote location anaesthesia
- Outline the problems in providing general anaesthesia for an adult in the MRI suite. (1/08)

Statistics and research
- What are the key objectives of an ethical review of a research project? (2/09)
- How is an appropriate sample size for a clinical trial determined? What are the ethical implications of using an inappropriate sample size? (1/09)
- Explain the terms sensitivity, specificity, positive predictive value and negative predictive value when applied to a diagnostic test. (2/08)
- Describe the advantages and disadvantages of multi-centre trials in anaesthesia research. (1/08)
- Discuss the ethical considerations in having a placebo group in a trial to evaluate a new analgesic. (2/07)
- Discuss ways in which you can decrease bias in a clinical trial for a new antihypertensive agent. (2/05)
- Discuss the value of case reports to anaesthetists in the era of evidence-based medicine. (1/05)

Transfusion medicine
- Outline the coagulation changes occurring from liver rupture requiring massive transfusion and how to minimise them. (1/09)
- Critically evaluate the role of recombinant factor VIIa in blood loss requiring massive transfusion in the trauma patient. (2/06)
- Compare the relative merits of gelatin-based intravenous solutions and dextran intravenous solutions. (1/05)
- Discuss the advantages and disadvantages of intraoperative blood salvage. (1/05)

Trauma anaesthesia
- Describe the principles of cerebral protection in a patient with an isolated closed head injury. (2/09)
- A woman suffers fractured sternum following blunt chest trauma. List the injuries to the heart that may be caused by this blunt trauma. In the absence of signs or symptoms of cardiac injury, list and justify screening investigations for cardiac injury you would perform. (2/07)
- Define circulatory shock. Categorise the causes of circulatory shock and give an example in each category. (2/07)
- Describe the principles of cerebral protection in a patient with an isolated closed head injury. (2/06)

Vascular anaesthesia

- List indications and contra-indications for the use of an intra-aortic balloon pump. Describe how its performance is optimised. (2/08)
- Describe cardiovascular changes which occur during clamping and unclamping the supra-renal aorta during AAA repair in a patient with normal ventricular function. Outline your strategies to maintain critical organ perfusion during these times. (2/06)
- Discuss the principles underlying the management of general anaesthesia for carotid endarterectomy. (1/06)

Welfare, consent and quality assurance issues

- Outline steps to ensure the safe introduction of elective paediatric surgery at your local private hospital. (1/09)
- In what circumstances is it permissible to permanently hand over responsibility for an anaesthetic, and how would you ensure this handover occurs safely? (2/08)
- What are the signs that may make you suspect opioid abuse in a colleague? Outline principles that should guide intervention. (2/08)
- Why is consent for a medical procedure necessary? What makes it valid? (1/07)
- Describe factors that contribute to intravenous drug errors in anaesthesia practice. Discuss methods available to reduce the incidence of such errors. (1/06)
- Discuss elements you consider important when obtaining consent for epidural analgesia in labour. (1/06)
- Discuss the purpose of a postoperative visit. (2/05)
- A patient asks you to administer an alternative medicine as part of their anaesthesia for total hip replacement. How would you respond to this? (2/05)
- A recovery nurse approaches you because of concern at the amount of opiates one of your trainees has been signing out for patients. What will be your priorities in addressing the nurse's concern? (1/05)

Chapter 4

The medical vivas

The worst time to have a heart attack is during a game of charades.
DEMETRI MARTIN

Overview

The medical vivas take place the day after the written examination, and consist of two 18-minute examination stations involving a clinical encounter with a real patient. The medical vivas evaluate candidates' ability to perform an appropriate preoperative assessment. Candidates must take a relevant history, perform a focused examination eliciting physical signs and review investigation results, allowing them to enter into a discussion of the pathophysiology and functional reserve of the patient in relation to the risks of anaesthesia.

Marks in this component of the exam are allocated for the appropriateness of the history-taking and whether key symptoms are elicited. Candidates are expected to listen to the patient and also respond to their non-verbal cues. In the examination stage, candidates are marked on an examination technique which is sequential and logical, and which elicits key signs. Professionalism is also judged, and candidates are expected to show patients respect, with concern for their comfort and modesty. Finally, an organised and efficient presentation of findings is expected; candidates must show good knowledge of the medical condition present and its implications for anaesthesia.

The medical viva seems to have changed subtly in its emphasis over the years. In the past it was purely medical history and examination without much anaesthetic flavour, but it is now more likely to include discussions about the anaesthetic implications of the condition. The candidate should be prepared for this. You are generally not expected to examine specific anaesthetic areas of interest, such as the airway, unless it is a specific problem with the condition. For example, the case of a patient with aortic stenosis undergoing cardiovascular examination would probably not require comment about their airway, whereas that of a patient with rheumatoid arthritis probably would.

Performance strategies

Many candidates find this component of the examination the most stressful, in both its preparation and its execution. In essence, this is what trainees spend their working lives doing, so why is this part of the exam so intimidating? Firstly, there is significant time pressure in the patient evaluation stations, and many candidates worry about being rushed and missing critical historical information or examination signs, evoking memories of difficult medical short cases performed in undergraduate examinations. This pressure has been relieved somewhat in recent years with the extension of the viva time to 18 minutes. Specific preparation for this section of the examination is often neglected as candidates concentrate on the sections of the written examination.

One of the most common criticisms of candidates is that their interrogation and examination techniques lack polish. Part of the reason for this is that most of us become used to a non-physician-like patient assessment which is not directed at a single organ system. We take significant and calculated shortcuts, often dictated by the time pressure of a large room of patients at a busy outpatient clinic. It is unusual for an anaesthetist to examine individual organ systems in turn.

It is therefore important to specifically practise for this part of the examination. Where possible, perform a single-system examination on preoperative patients to refresh any long-forgotten techniques and sequences. It is important to have a smooth examination technique for cardiovascular, respiratory, neurological and endocrine systems, and examination of the abdomen. Enlist the help of colleagues to find patients you can practise upon. Subject yourself to the scrutiny of your physician and intensivist colleagues in examination conditions as often as you can. Textbooks on physical examination, such as those by Talley and O'Connor (see Chapter 2 for details), are essential revision.

The only equipment you will need to bring with you to the medical vivas is a stethoscope. Before the day of the exam it is worth checking the patency of your stethoscope from the diaphragm to the earpieces, especially if it has lain idle for a period of time. Also remember to wash your hands before and after seeing each patient. This is commonsense, good hygiene and displays an appropriate degree of professionalism.

During the two-minute perusal time before the viva commences, write down the name and age of the patient, which will be provided on the door. A limited clinical history (which may include a list of medications) is often provided before you enter the room, and may offer some clues as to the clinical scenario to be encountered. It is important to concentrate on the instructions that have been provided very carefully, as your enquiries and examination will be directed towards a specific system or component thereof.

Candidates tend to employ one of two techniques in the medical vivas. The first and most common of these is to perform the history-taking and examination sequentially. The advantage of this approach is that it may be more familiar and comfortable for candidates. The second approach is to take the history and perform the examination simultaneously. This method is more efficient and allows for more information to be gleaned in the small amount of time allowed. It is technically more demanding, however, and trainees who plan to use this method will need to practise it many times. They must also be wary of missing important clues from the history or examination because of the distraction of performing both together.

The examiners' reports in the past have been scathing of candidates who have not shown good interpersonal skills with patients. You must always be friendly and polite, and listen carefully to what the patient has to say. Be respectful of their modesty during the examination process, and under no circumstances do anything that will be uncomfortable for the patient or hurt them. Always thank the patient before leaving them for the discussion. On rare occasions the viva examinations will enlist the use of inpatients who are very unwell, and whose condition may deteriorate during the exam itself. If your patient should become unwell/collapse/lose consciousness/arrest, then immediately discard the trappings of pretence of the examination and alert the examiner to the situation. Do what you can to help given the resources available to you.

Remember you have only eight or nine minutes to carry out your history and examination, so you must be focused in your approach. Always remember to ask about previous anaesthetics and a list of medications (if not provided earlier), and always try to ascertain the functional status of the patient and whether or not they are fully optimised. Patients are not instructed to withhold any information, and are often quite good at providing you with a succinct, relevant summary of their condition. It is perfectly acceptable to ask a patient what diagnosis they have been given, or what they have been led to understand about their condition.

In your examination of the patient it is important not to imagine signs that you think should be present. For example, a well-managed patient with a history of left ventricular failure may have a clear chest on auscultation.

When the discussion period commences, begin with a concise summary of the patient's history, functional reserve and examination findings, and, where possible, the relevance of these to any proposed anaesthesia and/or surgery. The examiners will then discuss management aspects of the case, or may provide you with the opportunity to ask for and review any investigations you think relevant. It is inevitable that such investigations will appear at this point; the majority of these will be electrocardiographs, chest X-rays, arterial blood gases, spirometry and haematology results. You can also expect to see cervical spine and abdominal plain films, CT scans and MRI scans; echocardiographical, pulmonary artery catheter and sleep study data occasionally appear.

You should have a systematic technique for reviewing ECGs and CXRs. Begin by outlining the process of your technique as you go. After doing this the first time, the examiner may ask you to simply comment on any obvious abnormality on subsequent results. Commonly encountered investigations are discussed further in Chapter 6.

Always be prepared to comment on the implications of any findings and their relevance to anaesthesia.

It should be reassuring to candidates that the pass rate for the medical viva component of the examination is very high, usually similar to that of the anaesthesia vivas. Again, the usefulness of practice cannot be overemphasised.

Some sample medical viva cases are presented here to give you an indication of the type of focused history and examination that may be required in the examination. Topics for discussion are also provided.

Patient assessment stations

1. The patient with aortic valve stenosis

Possible clinical scenario

Mrs I E, 64, is due to undergo elective femoral hernia repair. She presents with worsening shortness of breath when climbing stairs. Please take a relevant history and conduct an examination as you see fit.

Appropriate thoughts

Before you enter the room you should be focused on either a cardiac or respiratory cause to explain the symptom outlined here.

Ischaemic and/or valvular heart disease, or chronic lung disease, need to be uncovered early in the encounter to allow for a thorough directed history and examination.

First impressions

- Note whether the patient appears to be an inpatient (hospital pyjamas, wheelchair, oxygen) or an outpatient. This may provide clues as to the severity of the underlying disorder.
- Is the patient dyspnoeic at rest?

History

- Patients with aortic stenosis will usually be able to tell you the diagnosis or some variant thereof ('a squeaky, very exciting Antarctic valve' was told to one recent candidate).
- The classic triad of symptoms are angina, exertional dyspnoea and exertional syncope.
- Ask about the time-frame of evolution of symptoms (often latent period >30 years) and speed of progression recently.
- Is there a history of rheumatic fever? If so, you need to consider the possibility of co-existing mitral valve disease. If not, other causes are calcification of a bicuspid valve and degenerative calcific stenosis (common in the elderly).
- Assess the patient's exercise tolerance and functional reserve.
- Is there evidence of ventricular failure? Ask about orthopnoea, paroxysmal nocturnal dyspnoea and ankle swelling.
- Ask about other risk factors for coronary artery disease.
- What treatment options have been undertaken or planned?
- Obtain a list of medications, other medical conditions and allergies.

Physical examination

Position the patient at 45 degrees for cardiovascular examination and ask for the blood pressure (the examiners may make you take it yourself).

- Assess pulses for:
  - rate and rhythm
  - slow uptake or plateau carotid pulse
  - collapsing pulse (if concomitant significant aortic incompetence)
  - radio-radial and radiofemoral delay
- Assess jugular venous pressure (JVP)
- Examine the praecordium for:
  - previous cardiac surgical scars
  - displaced apex beat
  - hyperdynamic apex beat
  - aortic thrill (a sign of severity).
- Auscultate the chest:
  - Listen to the loudness of heart sounds and splitting
  - Is there a fourth heart sound?
  - Is there an ejection systolic murmur loudest in the second intercostal space radiating to neck (may be present throughout praecordium)? Listen for radiation throughout praecordium and/or axilla (if other murmurs suspected).

- Listen carefully for an early diastolic murmur in expiration with patient sitting forward (aortic regurgitation will often be present to some degree).
- Louder grade of murmur, later timing of peak intensity and soft or absent second heart sounds have been suggested as indicators of severity; such signs may be subtle and do not necessarily differentiate moderate and severe disease.
- Perform dynamic manoeuvres:
  - Leg raise or squat increases preload and makes the murmur louder.
  - Valsalva (decreased preload) and hand grip (increased afterload) should, in theory, make the murmur softer.
- Check lung fields for crepitations, and the lower limbs for oedema.

Useful statements

'Mrs E gives a history of angina and dyspnoea after climbing two flights of stairs, which has been associated with syncope on two occasions. Combined with the presence of a slow upstroke carotid pulse and mid-systolic murmur radiating to the neck, I believe she has significant aortic valve stenosis, which is most likely due to a calcified aortic valve. I would seek to investigate this further before embarking on the planned elective surgery.'

Investigations

- Echocardiography: check valve area, derived gradients across valve (mean and peak), which depend for their accuracy on the contractile state of the ventricle; check left and right ventricular function
- Chest X-ray: look for post-stenotic aortic dilatation, left ventricular hypertrophy
- ECG: check voltage criteria for left ventricular hypertrophy, left ventricular strain
- Cardiac catheterisation: assess measurement of pressure gradients, look for concomitant coronary artery disease (if surgery planned).

Topics for discussion

- Classification of severity of aortic stenosis based on valve area, transvalvular pressure gradient
- NYHA classification of perioperative risk: should surgery be cancelled?
- Options for treatment of aortic stenosis: when is surgery indicated?
- Options for anaesthesia for non-cardiac surgery
- Antibiotic prophylaxis
- Central neuraxial blockade and aortic stenosis
- Haemodynamic goals during non-cardiac surgery and how to achieve these
- Role for invasive monitoring: what are particular problems with pulmonary artery catheterisation?
- What are your priorities in the event of this patient sustaining a cardiac arrest?
- The ventricular pressure/volume relationship in aortic stenosis.

2. The patient with ischaemic heart disease

Possible clinical scenario

Mrs R C, aged 72, is due for right total hip replacement in 3 months' time. She has recently had worsening chest pain and was admitted to hospital last week. Please take a brief history and examine her cardiovascular system.

Appropriate thoughts

Acute-on-chronic myocardial ischaemia is the most likely cause for these symptoms. It is important to gain an impression of the severity of the disease when assessing the patient. In this situation it is also possible that the patient has suffered a myocardial infarct.

First impressions

- Is the patient an inpatient? Look for oxygen, intravenous therapy and/or drugs.
- Is she dyspnoeic at rest?
- Look for obvious bruising from venepuncture/arterial sites, which may indicate thrombolysis. Is there any obvious oedema?

History

- Determine the nature of the chest pain and whether it is typical of myocardial ischaemia.
- Always keep gastro-oesophageal reflux in mind as a differential diagnosis.
- What precipitated the admission to hospital?
- Has the patient had unstable angina (recent onset, worsening of previous angina, or symptoms at rest) or a myocardial infarct?
- Is there any history of dyspnoea, orthopnoea or paroxysmal nocturnal dyspnoea?
- What treatment did she receive (e.g. thrombolysis, cardiac catheterisation, stenting, stress test, echocardiography) and were there any complications (e.g. arrhythmias, failure, bleeding problems)? Has this resulted in a reduction in symptoms?
- Assess the patient's functional reserve (metabolic equivalents are useful): walking distance on the flat and uphill/on stairs. Assess other limitations to normal activities of daily living.
- Ask about cardiac risk factors and any efforts to control these:
  - diabetes
  - lipid profile
  - hypertension
  - smoking
  - family history
  - OCP/menopause
  - obesity.
- Obtain a list of all medications and any allergies.

Physical examination

Position the patient at 45 degrees for cardiovascular examination.

- Take note of any intravenous therapy they may be receiving.
- Ask to measure the blood pressure.
- Feel the pulse for rate and rhythm.
- Feel for radio-radial and radiofemoral delay.
- Examine the mouth for cyanosis.
- Assess the JVP for height and character and feel and auscultate the carotid pulses.
- Inspect the praecordium for surgical scars, visible apex beat and pacemakers.
- Assess the location and character of the apex beat and any praecordial thrills and parasternal impulses.

- Auscultate for:
  - first and second heart sounds
  - heart murmurs, especially infarct related VSD or mitral regurgitation
  - crepitations at the lung bases.
- Assess for the presence of peripheral oedema.

In a well-managed patient there may be surprisingly little to find on clinical examination.

Do not manufacture signs that are not present.

Useful statements

'Mrs C is currently an inpatient, having been admitted with unstable angina 1 week ago, with central chest pain radiating to her left arm at rest. She has a history of 15 years of stable angina, which had been treated with aspirin, beta blockers and calcium channel blockers. She underwent coronary angioplasty and stenting with resolution of her symptoms. She can currently walk 200 m on the flat before onset of dyspnoea.'

Investigations

- ECG (baseline and acute event if possible): comment on any arrhythmias, evidence of ischaemia or infarction. If infarct, ST segment elevation myocardial infarction (STEMI) or non-STEMI?
- Echocardiography
- Chest X-ray: signs of cardiomegaly, acute ventricular failure
- Cardiac catheterisation data.

Topics for discussion

- Cyclo-oxygenase (COX)-2 inhibitors and myocardial ischaemia
- Intraoperative monitoring for elective surgery
- Benefits of general vs regional techniques in patients with minimal cardiac reserve
- Justify your choice of anaesthesia for hip replacement surgery
- Intraoperative monitoring for myocardial ischaemia; use of transoesophageal echocardiography (TOE)
- Role of B-type natriuretic peptide in diagnosis and prognosis of myocardial injury
- Treatment of intraoperative ischaemia
- Timing of post-infarct elective surgery
- Timing of cardiac surgery; benefits of stenting versus coronary artery bypass grafting
- Management of patients with bare metal/drug-eluting stents, platelet inhibitors and elective surgery.

3. The patient with hypertension

Possible clinical scenario

Mr O T, 45, was due for elective varicose vein ligation, but cancelled because of high blood pressure. Please conduct a relevant history and examination.

Appropriate thoughts

On rare occasions the examiners may give you very specific information to focus your attention. In this case you should be considering causes of hypertension (remembering that over 90% of cases are essential hypertension), the possibility of co-existent cardiorespiratory disease, and the effect of hypertension on other organ systems.

First impressions
- Are characteristic features of a secondary cause of hypertension present? A spot diagnosis of Cushing's syndrome, acromegaly or myxoedema may lead to a modification of your approach.
- If the patient is an inpatient, this may be related to the investigation or treatment of hypertension, and again might raise suspicions of a secondary cause (e.g. renal artery stenosis, Conn's syndrome or phaeochromocytoma).

History
- Ask when the diagnosis of hypertension was made, and approximate readings in recent times. How high have readings been in the past?
- Is the patient aware of a diagnosis associated with their hypertension?
  - adrenal tumour
  - renal disease or renal artery stenosis
  - aortic coarctation
  - acromegaly
  - myxoedema
  - obstructive sleep apnoea.
- Ask about factors that contribute to essential hypertension:
  - alcohol
  - obesity
  - cigarette smoking
  - poor diet and exercise patterns.
- What treatment has the patient received for their hypertension and how successful has it been?
- Have there been any complications from the hypertension?
  - peripheral vascular disease
  - visual problems
  - strokes.

Physical examination
- Measure the patient's blood pressure lying and standing. Ask for measurements in each arm. Readings >140/>90 mmHg indicate the presence of hypertension.
- Carefully feel the peripheral pulses. It is appropriate to test for radio-radial delay and radiofemoral delay.
- Palpate and auscultate the carotid pulses. Ask to examine the fundi (you may be told the results of fundoscopic examination).
- Examine the chest and listen for murmurs, a fourth heart sound and evidence of left ventricular failure.
- Examine the abdomen for surgical scars, and feel for aortic aneurysms and renal masses, auscultate for renal bruits.

Useful statements
'Mr T is a 45-year-old gentleman who presented 6 months ago for elective surgery which was cancelled because of a blood pressure reading of 220/110 mmHg. He had suffered headaches and blurred vision for a month before this. Prior to this he

was in excellent health and received yearly check-ups with no problems recorded. This history suggests a secondary cause of his hypertension, and Mr T confirms that further investigation resulted in a diagnosis of Conn's syndrome for which he underwent laparoscopic right adrenalectomy last week. He is on no current medication.

'Examination today reveals a blood pressure of 110/70 mmHg in both arms with no postural drop. Cardiovascular system examination is otherwise unremarkable. Abdominal examination shows normal healing of laparoscopic port scars and no other abnormality.'

Investigations

- Urea and electrolytes: preoperative values for the classical features of Conn's syndrome (note that Cushing's syndrome can also cause hypokalaemia), renal disease
- BSL and lipid profile
- ECG: voltage criteria for left ventricular hypertrophy
- Urinalysis for blood, protein and collection for catecholamines
- Chest X-ray
- Other imaging studies based on clinical suspicion (adrenal tumours, renal artery stenosis).

Topics for discussion

- Causes of secondary hypertension
- Threshold for cancelling elective surgery and further management of hypertensive patients; what are the likely intraoperative problems to be expected?
- Classes of antihypertensive drugs
- Perioperative management of patients with phaeochromocytoma
- Causes and management of hypertensive crises.

4. The patient with a permanent pacemaker/implantable defibrillator

Possible clinical scenario

Mr T A, aged 75, presents for transurethral resection of the prostate. He has had recent attacks of dizziness and palpitations. Please take a history and conduct a cardiovascular examination.

Appropriate thoughts

While concomitant cerebrovascular disease is a possibility, the likely focus of this case is cardiovascular, specifically cardiac arrhythmias and/or valvular lesions.

First impressions

- Is the patient an inpatient? This may suggest a recurring or chronic cause with recent management with which the patient may be familiar.
- It is unlikely the examiners will recruit an unwell inpatient with an unstable life-threatening arrhythmia.
- A well-looking, happy outpatient may reflect successful treatment.

History

A succinct history may well provide you with most of the information you need.
- Outline the time-frame of the presenting symptoms.
  - Was there any associated chest pain?
  - How often and under what circumstances (e.g. exertion) did the symptoms occur?
  - Can the patient tap out the palpitations; were they rapid/regular/irregular?
  - What exactly did the dizziness entail?
- Rapid irregular palpitations suggest atrial fibrillation.
- Regular palpitations suggest supraventricular or ventricular tachycardia.
- Heart block and sick sinus syndrome are less likely in the presence of palpitations.
- Detail any history of previous heart disease, especially ischaemia or prior cardiac surgery.
- Determine if there is a family history of cardiac disease or arrhythmias (e.g. hypertrophic obstructive cardiomyopathy, congenital long QT syndromes).
- Ask for details of treatment received:
  - Was treatment in the emergency department or subsequently as an inpatient?
  - Were physical manoeuvres (e.g. carotid sinus massage) employed?
  - Were any drugs used? (Patients may remember treatment with adenosine.)
  - Has the patient undergone cardiac catheterisation, electrophysiology studies or cardioversion?
- The presence of a pacemaker suggests an underlying bradyarrhythmia or biventricular failure. The presence of an automatic implanted cardioverter–defibrillator (AICD) suggests VT, VF or prolonged QT syndrome.
- For pacemakers and AICDs, ask when they were put in and if there have been any problems since. Does the patient carry a pacemaker card with the programming details?
- How often is the device tested and when was this last done?
- Are symptoms entirely controlled? How often does the DC shock go off?
- Ask about functional reserve pre- and post-treatment. Obtain a list of all medications.

Physical examination
- Perform your normal cardiovascular examination, focusing specifically on the pulse rate, rhythm and character.
- Note the presence of scars, indicating previous surgery, and the presence of a pacemaker or AICD device.

Useful statements

'Mr A is an elderly gentleman who presented 6 months ago with dizziness and rapid regular palpitations on a background of ischaemic heart disease treated with CABG 5 years ago. These symptoms occurred on moderate exertion and on one occasion included a syncopal event, resulting in his hospitalisation and admission to coronary care, where he was treated with intravenous therapy and underwent subsequent cardiac catheterisation and electrophysiological studies. He was fitted with an AICD device and has experienced DC shocks on four occasions since. His exercise tolerance has improved and he can walk 1 km on the flat with no dyspnoea, chest pain or other symptoms. Examination shows him to be in sinus rhythm, 84 beats per minute, with an obvious implanted device in the left sub-clavicular area. Cardiovascular examination was otherwise unremarkable. I suspect that Mr A was suffering episodes of VT, and that he has a device with overdrive pacing and DC cardioversion facilities. I would seek further elucidation from his cardiologist before embarking on elective surgery.'

Investigations
- ECG: ask for this pre-treatment if possible: QT, SVT, VT, heart block and its variations, atrial fibrillation
- Serum electrolytes: potassium, magnesium
- Echocardiography
- Chest X-ray: position of the device and location of electrodes
- Catheterisation data/EPS data
- Ask for a report of the most recent check of the device.

Topics for discussion
- Types of pacemaker/defibrillator and their classification (see Tables 4.1 and 4.2)
- Use of biventricular pacing in the treatment of cardiac failure
- Hazards of using magnets with implanted cardiac devices
- Indications for pacemaker insertion
- Indications for AICD insertion
- Management of elective surgery and pacemakers: diathermy, disabling functions
- What contingency plans would you have in place if the device failed?

TABLE 4.1 The North American Society of Pacing and Electrophysiology (NASPE) and British Pacing and Electrophysiology Group (BPEG) Generic Pacemaker Coding System

Letter position	I	II	III	IV	V
Category	Chamber paced	Chamber sensed	Response to sensing	Rate modulation	Multisite pacing
Letters	O = none	O = none	O = none	O = none	O = none
	A = atrium	A = atrium	T = triggered	R = rate modulation	A = atrium
	V = ventricle	V = ventricle	I = inhibited		V = ventricle
	D = dual	D = dual	D = dual (T+I)		D = dual

Source: AD Bernstein, AJ Camm, RD Fletcher, et al. The NASPE/BPEG generic pacemaker code for antibradyarrhythmia and adaptive-rate pacing and antitachyarrhythmia devices. Pacing and Clinical Electrophysiology 1987; 10:794–9.

TABLE 4.2 The North American Society of Pacing and Electrophysiology (NASPE) and British Pacing and Electrophysiology Group (BPEG) Defibrillator Coding System

Letter position	I	II	III	IV
Category	Chamber shocked	Antitachycardia pacing chamber	Antitachycardia detection	Pacing chamber
Letters	O = none	O = none	E = electrogram	O = none
	A = atrium	A = atrium	H = haemodynamic	A = atrium
	V = ventricle	V = ventricle		V = ventricle
	D = dual	D = dual		D = dual

Source: AD Bernstein, JC Daubert, RD Fletcher et al. The revised NASPE/BPEG generic code for antibradycardia, adaptive rate, and multisite pacing. Pacing and Clinical Electrophysiology 2002; 25:260–4.

5. The patient with peripheral vascular disease

Possible clinical scenario

Mr E T, 65, has suffered worsening leg pain for a number of years. Please take a history and conduct an appropriate cardiovascular examination.

Appropriate thoughts

• You should be alerted to a possible vascular cause, although from the given history it is possible the patient suffers from a chronic pain syndrome.
• It is important to assess risk factors and co-morbidities.
• Functional assessment of vascular patients is critically important.

First impressions

• Is the patient an inpatient? There may be evidence of recent limb or abdominal surgery.
• Are there any obvious previous limb amputations?

History

• A history of the site, nature and progression of limb pain is important. Patients with peripheral vascular disease can typically walk a fixed distance before needing to rest from claudication. This distance may shorten over time until pain is present even at rest.
• Concomitant features may include limb swelling, ulceration and gangrene.
• Note that a very active patient with mild disease may suffer more discomfort than a sedentary patient with more severe disease.
• Ask about risk factors for atherosclerosis: hyperlipidaemia, obesity, smoking, age, diabetes and hypertension. Note that peripheral vascular disease may also encompass aneurysmal disease caused by rarer conditions such as Marfan's and Ehlers-Danlos syndromes.
• Atherosclerosis may affect the entire vascular tree, so it is important to ask about symptoms of cerebrovascular insufficiency, renal dysfunction and ischaemic heart disease. The limitation of functional capacity from claudication may mask symptoms of coronary artery disease (which is significant in up to 75% of patients with peripheral vascular disease).

Physical examination
- Examine the legs looking for skin integrity, asymmetry, pallor and capillary refill. Examine all peripheral pulses on both sides.
- Measure the blood pressure (or ask for the results) in both arms and both legs. The ankle/brachial index is the highest systolic blood pressure from the dorsalis pedis or posterior tibial artery divided by the systolic blood pressure measured at the brachial artery; a value of <0.6 may indicate severe lower limb ischaemia.
- Examine the heart and lung fields for valve lesions, signs of congestive heart failure and evidence of chronic lung disease from smoking.
- Palpate and auscultate the carotid arteries for a thrill or bruit.
- Palpate the abdomen for the presence of an aortic aneurysm.

Useful statements
'Mr T is currently an inpatient being treated for a wound infection following right-sided femoro-popliteal bypass grafting 8 days ago. His risk factors for peripheral vascular disease include a 40-pack-year history of cigarette smoking, raised cholesterol and systemic hypertension. He has suffered intermittent claudication for 5 years, with the claudication distance being steady at 200 m walking on the flat, until this year when the distance dramatically decreased to around 25 m. He also reports suffering pain at rest that wakes him from sleep. He also has a history of stable angina for which he is on medical treatment, including beta-blocker therapy. His surgery was conducted with general anaesthesia and was unremarkable from the patient's perspective.

'On examination his surgical wounds are covered, with a hospital request to keep them so. There is no sign of obvious surrounding infection. Both dorsalis pedis pulses are palpable and strong. I cannot feel a left posterior tibial pulse, but it is present on the right side. Capillary refill is sluggish in both feet. Brachial blood pressure is 150/80; the calculated preoperative right ankle:brachial index from the information given to me is 0.5, a possible indication of severe lower limb ischaemia. Heart sounds are normal and other peripheral pulses are present. Auscultation of the carotid arteries reveals no bruits.'

Investigations
- The functional severity of claudication can be assessed using the Rutherford Standard exercise protocol (treadmill walking for 5 minutes at 3 km/h up a 2% incline)
- Limb imaging investigations include Doppler ultrasound, magnetic resonance angiography and dye angiography
- Preoperative testing prior to revascularisation should include respiratory function tests, ECG, chest X-ray, baseline bloods and echocardiography if aortic disease or symptomatic coronary artery disease
- In this patient, postoperative full blood count and wound microbiology, culture and sensitivities, and possibly blood cultures would also be of interest.

Topics for discussion
- Regional anaesthesia and management of anticoagulation
- Institution of beta-blocker therapy to decrease cardiac risk
- Techniques of regional anaesthesia for carotid endarterectomy
- Management of aortic cross-clamping
- Pre-emptive analgesia/pain management for amputation.

6. The patient with chronic obstructive pulmonary disease

Possible clinical scenario

Mr I T is a 54-year-old man with wheeze and shortness of breath on exertion. He is scheduled for semi-elective laparoscopic hernia repair. Please take a history and examine his respiratory system.

Appropriate thoughts

This combination of symptoms may steer your thinking to respiratory rather than cardiac pathophysiology, although it is important to remember that the two often co-exist.

If so, you should seek to determine the contribution of each to the underlying problem. Likely respiratory causes might be chronic bronchitis, emphysema, asthma, bronchiectasis and lung carcinoma, all of which can be elucidated on history and examination.

Consider the possible implications of any underlying pathology on the proposed surgery.

First impressions

- Is the patient dyspnoeic or cyanosed at rest?
- Are they using supplemental oxygen?
- Is the patient cachectic, nicotine-stained or obviously clubbed?
- You may not be able to see inside a sputum cup as you walk in, but its presence may give you a clue to a diagnosis (a polystyrene cup in the room may also contain the examiner's coffee).

History

- Ask specifically about the duration and severity of presenting symptoms.
- Ask also about cough and sputum production, and any other symptoms that may be present.
- What is the diagnosis of the patient's problem?
- Are there any precipitants or factors which worsen the condition?
- Is the patient using home oxygen? How many hours a day?
- Determine any restriction on function and reserve:
  - metabolic equivalent exercise tolerated
  - walking distance on flat and uphill/stairs
  - limitations to normal activities of daily living.
- Determine underlying causes:
  - duration and magnitude of cigarette smoking
  - occupational exposure (e.g. asbestos)
  - infections (e.g. tuberculosis)
  - genetic illnesses (alpha-1-anti-trypsin deficiency).
- Elucidate current treatment of the patient's symptoms:
  - home oxygen
  - bronchodilators
  - antibiotics
  - steroid therapy
  - physiotherapy
  - recent admissions to hospital, including intensive care/ventilation episodes.
- Ask about any recent surgery and any complications that may have occurred.

It is easiest to examine the respiratory system with the patient sitting up.
- Examine the patient peripherally for cyanosis and clubbing (which will usually indicate co-existent disease, e.g. carcinoma, fibrosis or chronic infection). Warm peripheries and a bounding pulse may indicate carbon dioxide retention. Pulsus paradoxus may be present.
- Consider the patient's pattern of breathing, respiratory rate and effort, including the use of accessory muscles, intercostal recession and tracheal tug.
- Is the patient centrally cyanosed?
- Ask the patient to breathe in deeply and breathe out as rapidly and completely as possible. Look for wheeze and prolonged expiration time beyond a few seconds.
- Posterior chest:
  - examine for overinflation, scars
  - palpate for reduced expansion
  - percussing the chest may be of use if you suspect the possibility of localised infection or a pleural effusion
  - auscultate the chest to evaluate breath sounds in terms of quality and symmetry, and any adventitious sounds (crepitations and wheezes), and whether these change with coughing.
- Anterior chest:
  - inspection
  - chest expansion
  - percussion
  - auscultation.

Position the patient at 45 degrees and palpate the apex beat and look for a parasternal heave suggestive of right ventricular hypertrophy. Listen for a loud pulmonary component of the second heart sound.

In a patient whose airflow limitation is not severe, or extremely well-managed, there may be few clinical signs present on the day of the examination.

'Mr T is a middle-aged gentleman who has moderately severe chronic obstructive pulmonary disease, secondary to a 20-pack-year history of cigarette smoking, which is ongoing. He has recently been hospitalised for 1 week following an infective exacerbation of his condition. He suffers functional limitation from his condition and is unable to walk up more than one flight of stairs or 400 m on level ground without resting. He currently uses nebulised salbutamol approximately four times a day at home.

'On examination he is cachectic with nicotine-staining of his fingers and is peripherally cyanosed. He is not centrally cyanosed. There is limited chest wall expansion and reduced breath sounds globally, with expiratory wheeze present especially in the lower lung zones. His condition is not optimised for the proposed surgery and I would seek further investigations and instigate a management strategy prior to considering him for general anaesthesia.'

- Pulse oximetry on room air is a useful test
- Spirometry: restrictive/obstructive changes and effect of bronchodilators (changes of 15% in FEV_1 are considered significant), diffusion capacity for

carbon monoxide (DLCO) is reduced in emphysema, peak flow rates, flow–volume loops
- Chest X-ray: look for hyperinflation, infection
- ABG on room air: respiratory failure if pO_2 <50 mmHg, or pCO_2 >50 mmHg
- Full blood count: look for polycythaemia, increased Hb
- ECG: evidence of right ventricular hypertrophy, concomitant ischaemic heart disease.

Topics for discussion
- Strategies for optimisation of chronic airways limitation prior to surgery: role of outpatient clinics, respiratory physicians, exercise regimens and physiotherapy
- Smoking cessation and anaesthesia: timing and consequences
- Pneumoperitoneum and pulmonary consequences
- Surgery for severe emphysema: criteria for suitability and preoperative evaluation
- Choice of laparoscopic versus open surgical technique in this patient
- Strategies for intraoperative ventilation
- Management of the patient who fails extubation at the end of surgery.

7. The patient with pulmonary fibrosis

Possible clinical scenario
Mr T T is a 68-year-old former roofing worker who has been admitted to hospital with worsening shortness of breath. He is normally on home oxygen. Please take a brief history and examine his respiratory system.

Appropriate thoughts
From the history and examination request a pulmonary disease is likely, keeping in mind the possibility of concomitant right-sided cardiac disease/cor pulmonale. Perhaps a clue to the diagnosis lies in the occupational history.

First impressions
- Dyspnoea, cyanosis and oxygen therapy are all likely, and the patient may have obvious clubbing.
- Cachexia may be a sign of underlying malignancy.

History
- Where the diagnosis is known this will usually be forthcoming, especially in the case of occupational industrial dust disease. Determine the nature, severity and duration of exposure.
- Ask about age of onset of the disease and symptom progression, concentrating on functional limitations/exercise tolerance.
- Is there any history of smoking?
- Have systemic illnesses causing chronic lung disease been excluded, e.g. rheumatoid arthritis, systemic lupus, ankylosing spondylitis, scleroderma, polyarteritis, sarcoidosis, other autoimmune disease?
- Is there any history of pulmonary infection, e.g. tuberculosis, viral infection, fungal infection?

- Take a medication history (bleomycin, nitrofurantoin, amiodarone, methotrexate among others can cause interstitial lung disease).
- Discuss current treatment.
- Patients suffering from asbestosis are at increased risk of pleural plaque formation, bronchial carcinoma (especially if smokers) and malignant mesothelioma.

Physical examination
- Look for clubbing, central and peripheral cyanosis.
- Determine respiratory rate, look for use of accessory muscles.
- Percussion note may be dull over areas of pleural thickening/effusion/mesothelioma.
- Auscultate for fine inspiratory crepitations and wheeze.
- Look for signs of pulmonary hypertension/right ventricular hypertrophy (parasternal heave, loud pulmonary component of second heart sound).

Useful statements
'Mr T is a gentleman with respiratory impairment from known severe pulmonary fibrosis of 6 years. This is believed to be due to occupational asbestos exposure; he worked for more than 20 years in a grinding room of untreated boards with no respiratory protection or clothing decontamination facility. He has been on home oxygen therapy 12 hours per day for 3 years. He is unable to walk across the room without becoming short of breath. He was a heavy cigarette smoker between the ages of 15 and 35, after which time he quit. He was admitted to hospital 5 days ago with worsening shortness of breath and haemoptysis. He is due for a CT-guided biopsy of a lesion detected on chest X-ray and CT scanning, which his attending doctors fear may be malignant.

'On examination he is receiving oxygen via nasal prongs at 4 L/min. He was happy to attempt to talk while on room air, but rapidly became short of breath, unable to speak in sentences and dramatically centrally cyanosed, at which point we paused for him to put the oxygen back on. He is obviously clubbed and cachectic. His respiratory rate is 24 per minute. Chest auscultation reveals widespread, fine inspiratory crackles throughout both lung fields. He has no palpable cervical lymphadenopathy. There is no parasternal heave and heart sounds were normal.'

Investigations
- Respiratory function tests will typically show a restrictive pattern and reduced DLCO
- Chest X-ray may show pulmonary infiltrates, enlarged right ventricle, pleural plaques, pleural effusion, carcinoma
- Arterial blood gases
- ECG – evidence of right-sided hypertrophy/strain, right axis deviation, P pulmonale.

Topics for discussion
- Differential diagnosis of pulmonary infiltrates/fibrosis
- What is the role of preoperative echocardiography should such a patient present for emergency repair of an incarcerated hernia?
- What anaesthetic techniques would you employ in that circumstance, and why?

8. The patient with diabetes

Possible clinical scenario

Mr F R, 43, has recently undergone debridement of lower leg ulcers. Please take a brief history and examine the patient as you see fit.

Appropriate thoughts

- The history given in the scenario should lead you to a consideration of a patient with either peripheral vascular disease, diabetes mellitus, or both.
- Remember that diabetic patients are always available, so they commonly make an appearance in the medical vivas.
- Early questioning on the nature of the ulcers and surgery should point you in the right direction.

First impressions

Clues may be present as to the severity of any co-morbidities.
- Is the patient unwell and wheelchair-bound or an obvious outpatient?
- Are there any previous limb amputations?
- A general impression of the patient's weight may also be useful.

History

- Ask about the cause of the ulcers and any previous episodes of ulceration/ debridement.
- Determine whether the patient has type I or type II diabetes, and at what age it was diagnosed.
- Record the patient's hypoglycaemic regimen, including dietary control, oral hypoglycaemics and insulin: what type, how much and when?
- Determine the adequacy of control: how often is BSL measured and what is the pattern of results; has HbA1c been measured, and if so what was the result?
- Have there been any symptoms of hyperglycaemia (admissions with DKA, ongoing polyuria and thirst with weight loss) or episodes of hypoglycaemia (dizziness, loss of consciousness, sweats, seizures): if so, under what circumstances?

Importantly, determine the presence or absence of major co-morbidities:
- Cardiovascular:
  - ischaemic heart disease (including silent ischaemic episodes)
  - exercise tolerance
  - claudication
  - transient ischaemic attacks/stroke
  - hypertension.
- Nervous system:
  - peripheral neuropathy
  - autonomic neuropathy (fainting when standing, dizziness, erectile dysfunction).
- Vision:
  - lens and retinal disease.
- Renal system:
  - dysuria/nocturia
  - oedema
  - renal dysfunction or failure.

Obtain a history of other previous operations, diseases, drugs and allergies.

Physical examination

You may be directed towards a specific system.

- Ask for the patient's weight, BSL and blood pressure, standing and supine. (You may be invited to measure the blood pressure.)
- Position the patient for cardiovascular examination.
- Assess peripheral circulation:
  - temperature
  - capillary refill of peripheries
  - peripheral pulses: carotid, radial, femoral, popliteal, dorsalis pedis and posterior tibial.
- Inspect skin for ulceration and infection.
- Test sensation for peripheral neuropathy.
- Postural hypotension (fall of >30/20 mmHg on standing from supine position) may be an indicator of autonomic neuropathy, as may tachycardia at rest.
- Examination of the eyes is useful, including assessment of visual acuity, lens opacification and fundoscopy for haemorrhages, exudates and vessel proliferation. Ask to perform fundoscopy – the examiners may tell you the relevant findings.
- Examine the chest for co-existing cardiac disease (e.g. cardiomegaly) and auscultate the lung fields.
- Assess the patient's airway as you normally would (long-standing poor control may lead to a 'stiff joint syndrome' and increased incidence of intubation difficulties).

Useful statements

'Mr R has long-standing type II diabetes which is well controlled on his current oral hypoglycaemics, as evidenced by tight BSL control and reportedly low HbA1c. He does, however, have several end-organ complications of his disease, including autonomic neuropathy (as evidenced by a resting heart rate of 110 beats per minute and a postural drop in lying to standing blood pressure from 140/90 mmHg to 100/50 mmHg), peripheral neuropathy, absent peripheral pulses to palpation below the knee and vascular compromise resulting in ulceration and infection of his feet.'

Investigations

- Full blood count, random and fasting blood glucose, HbA1c, urea and electrolytes
- Urinalysis for glucose and protein
- Chest X-ray
- ECG: look for signs of ischaemia, QT variability.

Topics for discussion

- Perioperative management of BSL/oral drugs and insulin
- Classification of types of insulin
- Advantages/disadvantages of spinal vs general anaesthesia for lower limb debridement
- How to construct a sliding scale of insulin; advantages/disadvantages of subcutaneous versus intravenous scales
- Mechanism of action of: sulphonylureas, metformin, alpha-glucosidase inhibitors, thiazolidinediones
- Importance of intraoperative patient positioning
- Diagnosis and management of diabetic ketoacidosis
- Features of hyperosmolar nonketotic coma.

9. The patient with thyroid disease

Possible clinical scenario

Mrs S I, 57, has had recent weight loss. Please take a history and examine her head and neck.

Appropriate thoughts

Hyperthyroidism is the most likely explanation for the presenting symptom and examination request. Keep other possible causes (e.g. malignancy) in mind.

First impressions

- Does the patient have the characteristic facies of thyrotoxicosis? Is there an obvious goitre?
- Is there a glass of water nearby (suggesting sipping by patient during previous examination)?

History

- Ask about the history of weight loss: how much and over what time period?
- Does the patient have a diagnosis for their condition? How long has this been present?
- If you suspect hyperthyroidism as a cause, ask about other symptoms:
  - anxiety
  - palpitations
  - tremor
  - heat intolerance
  - fatigue
  - eye problems
  - sweating
  - diarrhoea, vomiting.
- If a goitre is present, ask about airway symptoms:
  - positional dyspnoea (suggesting retrosternal extension)
  - dysphagia
  - stridor
  - engorgement of head and neck veins; epistaxis
  - hoarseness/stridor (recurrent laryngeal nerve involvement).
- What treatment is the patient receiving?
- Ask about any associated diseases, previous operations and current treatment.

Physical examination

- Examine the eyes for lid retraction, lid lag, exophthalmos and conjunctivitis (which suggest Graves' disease).
- Inspect the neck and any possible thyroid swelling by getting the patient to take sips of water (a thyroid mass will rise with the larynx). See if you can see an inferior border to the mass.
- Look for prominent veins in the neck and upper chest.
- Palpate the neck from in front and behind, feeling the size and consistency of any swelling.
- It is important to locate the position of the trachea.

- Listen over the neck for a possible bruit, and ask the patient to raise their arms over their head, looking for congestion in the superior caval distribution (Pemberton's sign).
- While in the vicinity, assess the patient's airway as you normally would.

Useful statements

'Mrs I is currently an inpatient, undergoing investigation for signs and symptoms of hyperthyroidism. She has an 8-week history of 10 kg weight loss, palpitations, heat intolerance and dry eyes, with easy fatiguability causing absence from work. On examination she has a pronounced thyroid stare, exophthalmos and conjunctivitis, and a smooth diffuse swelling in the neck consistent with an enlarged thyroid. There are no signs of retrosternal extension, recurrent laryngeal nerve involvement or thoracic inlet obstruction. These findings are most consistent with a diagnosis of Graves' disease.'

Investigations

- Thyroid function tests: thyroid stimulating hormone (TSH), tri-iodothyronine (T3), thyroxine (T4), free concentration T4, T3 resin uptake, radioactive iodine scan
- CT scan
- ECG.

Topics for discussion

- Differential diagnosis of hyperthyroidism
- Pharmacological management of hyperthyroidism: carbimazole, propylthiouracil, beta-blockers
- Manifestations and treatment of thyroid storm
- Anaesthetic technique for thyroidectomy
- Diagnosis and management of postoperative hypocalcaemia
- Management of postoperative haematoma.

10. The patient with pituitary disease

Possible clinical scenario

Mr A E is a 55-year-old man who presented with headaches and visual disturbance for investigation, and is now booked on your elective neurosurgical list. Please take a history and examine the patient's visual field with the equipment provided, along with any other examination as you see fit.

Appropriate thoughts

The combination of presenting problems should suggest intracranial pathology somewhere along the visual pathway from the optic nerve to the occipital cortex. The possibility of a lesion near the optic chiasm should trigger some memories.

First impressions

- Patients with acromegaly secondary to a growth hormone secreting pituitary adenoma have characteristic facies with a large supraorbital ridge producing frontal 'bossing', a large, square, prognathic jaw, macroglossia and often

widely spaced teeth (the disease is sometimes first detected on dental examination).
- The voice may be hoarse from laryngeal tissue growth.
- Hands and feet (the peripheral or acral components) are typically broad and spade-like, such that the acromegalic handshake is encompassing, moist and doughy.

History

- Onset of bony and soft tissue changes is insidious and can go unnoticed for considerable time. Patients often cease to wear rings, and their shoe size often increases.
- Headache and visual disturbances are common presenting complaints.
- Paraesthesiae and arthralgias are common; up to 50% of patients may have carpal tunnel syndrome.
- There is a strong association with obstructive sleep apnoea; ask about: snoring, gasping, fatigue, irritability, daytime somnolence. (See subsequent scenario.)
- Patients may have cardiomyopathy and symptoms of left ventricular dysfunction.
- There is a tenuous association between acromegaly and colonic polyps and carcinoma.
- Ask about medications taken (octreotide, bromocriptine, cabergoline) and any side effects (orthostatic hypotension may occur with dopamine analogues such as bromocriptine).
- Is any radiotherapy planned? (Surgery is often a first-line option.)
- Ask about symptoms of diabetes. (Glucose intolerance is common.)

Physical examination

- Physical features, as described above, may lead to an immediate diagnosis.
- Spend some time evaluating the airway, as acromegalic features may predispose the patient to difficulties with bag and mask ventilation, and intubation.
- The classic visual field defect is a bitemporal hemianopia (central optic nerve fibres decussate at the optic chiasm near the sella), but a wide variety of field defects may be encountered.
- It is prudent to conduct a cardiovascular examination looking for signs of congestive cardiac failure and hypertension. There is an increased risk of vascular and ischaemic heart disease and stroke.
- Examine the abdomen for organomegaly.
- Multinodular goitre may be present.

Useful statements

'Mr E was diagnosed with acromegaly 7 weeks ago after presenting to his GP with headaches and reporting two traffic accidents where he sideswiped parked cars he did not see. A visiting relative also noticed a change in his appearance. On reflection, Mr E concedes noticing his shoe size has increased from 9 to 11 over a period of many months. He also reports suffering arthritic pains in most joints, and symptoms of snoring and daytime somnolence suggestive of sleep apnoea.

'On examination he has characteristic facies and hands of acromegaly. He has a large tongue, splayed teeth, an inter-incisor distance of 2 cm and a Mallampati score of 3 on airway examination. Visual field examination reveals a bitemporal hemianopia more extensive in the left visual field. There are no signs of respiratory or cardiac disease.

'He is scheduled for trans-sphenoidal hypophysectomy in 2 weeks' time.'

Investigations
- The diagnosis is usually confirmed by an increased assay of insulin-like growth factor IGF-1; prolactin levels may also be increased. Diagnosis can also be confirmed by failure of growth hormone suppression by glucose tolerance test.
- Other baseline tests of anterior pituitary function include assays of cortisol, thyroxine and gonadal hormones.
- While skull X-ray may show an enlarged sella, magnetic resonance imaging is the modality of choice. Pituitary adenomas appear hypodense on T1-weighted images and show less enhancement with gadolinium than surrounding tissue.
- Preoperative testing should include blood glucose measurement, ECG and echocardiography when concomitant cardiac disease is suspected.

Topics for discussion
- Management of a potentially difficult airway
- Complications of surgery: CSF rhinorrhoea, diabetes insipidus; how are they managed?
- Patient positioning for surgery: neurosurgical requirements, peripheral nerve protection.

11. The patient with morbid obesity/obstructive sleep apnoea

Possible clinical scenario
Mr L E, who is 40 years of age, recently underwent a laparoscopic gastric-banding operation. Please assess him as you see fit.

Appropriate thoughts
- Anticipate the obese patient.
- Consider the possible complications of obesity and how they may impact upon anaesthetic management.
- A patient scheduled for weight-reduction surgery will often talk happily and openly about their condition, but a degree of sensitivity is still required.

First impressions
- You will rapidly form an impression as to the magnitude of the patient's obesity.
- There may be evidence of concomitant disease (e.g. hypothyroidism or dyspnoea at rest).
- If the patient is an inpatient it is unlikely to be because of the recent surgery unless there were complications. (Patients are normally discharged around day 2.)

History
- Determine the patient's weight and height and calculate their body mass index (kg/m^2).
- Ask about any recent weight loss or gain, and over what time period changes have occurred, including any other therapies attempted prior to surgery.

- How has the patient's size impacted on their daily living and work?
- Ask the patient if he was made aware of any problems with the operation or anaesthetic.
- Ask about co-morbidities linked to obesity, specifically:
  - hypertension
  - hyperlipidaemia
  - type II diabetes
  - coronary artery disease
  - hypothyroidism
  - stroke
  - congestive cardiac failure
  - dysrhythmias
  - reflux
  - obstructive sleep apnoea.
- Patients with obstructive sleep apnoea may report a constellation of symptoms, including:
  - snoring
  - apnoea
  - choking
  - gasping
  - frequent awakening
  - daytime sleepiness
  - fatigue
  - irritability
  - defects in attention and memory
  - depression.
- Ask about how the diagnosis was made (usually on polysomnography) and whether the patient uses a continuous positive airway pressure (CPAP) device, and if so, how this has helped.
- Assess how the sleep apnoea has impacted on the patient's lifestyle, work and family.

Physical examination

- Determine the BMI, if you have not worked it out already.
- The airway should be carefully assessed, including mouth opening and Mallampati score, and any limitation of neck movement. Neck circumference has been proposed as an indicator of difficult intubation.
- Assess the blood pressure and perform cardiovascular examination, in particular looking for evidence of right ventricular hypertrophy and pulmonary hypertension.
- Listen to the lung fields.
- Examine the abdomen including the recent surgical scars. Feel for hepatomegaly (which may be difficult). Locate the subcutaneous reservoir for the gastric band, looking for signs of infection at the site.

Investigations

- Pulse oximetry on room air may be a good indicator of underlying pulmonary pathology
- Spirometry – assess for restrictive lung defect
- ABG – especially if low oxygen saturation on room air

- ECG – may show right-sided cardiac complications (right ventricular hypertrophy, right axis deviation) of sleep apnoea, left ventricular hypertrophy, arrhythmias
- Chest X-ray – look for advanced cardiac disease.
- Echocardiography – look for ventricular hypertrophy, contractility, pulmonary pressure (may need transoesophageal echo for adequate study).
- Polysomnography results.

Useful statements

'Mr E is a 40-year-old gentleman who has suffered from obesity for at least 20 years. He underwent laparoscopic gastric banding 2 weeks ago, prior to which he weighed 170 kg, which in conjunction with his height of 170 cm gives him a body mass index of 59. He has lost 10 kg since the surgery and appears well motivated. As well as his problem of morbid obesity, he was diagnosed with obstructive sleep apnoea 2 years ago, underwent sleep studies and has been using nocturnal CPAP, which has relieved his symptoms of snoring, daytime somnolence and fatigue. On examination of his airway I note that he has good neck movement in all directions, a Mallampati score of 3 with a normal thyromental distance and inter-incisor distance. His blood pressure is normal, and there were no signs of pulmonary hypertension or right-sided cardiac failure.'

Topics for discussion

- Metabolic syndrome
- Obesity hypoventilation syndrome
- Risk of reflux and aspiration; use of histamine receptor and proton blockers
- Intravenous access in obese patients
- Suitability of obese patients for day surgery
- Preoperative benefits of CPAP for obstructive sleep apnoea/obesity hypoventilation syndrome
- Pharmacokinetics in obesity
- Patient positioning
- Airway management
- Monitoring
- Problems of pneumoperitoneum in this patient
- Analgesia and obstructive sleep apnoea.

12. The patient with a spinal injury

Possible clinical scenario

Mrs I H is wheelchair-bound and due to undergo check rigid cystoscopy. Please conduct a history and relevant neurological examination.

Appropriate thoughts

You should be alert to the possibility of central nervous system or neuromuscular disease.

First impressions

- Does the patient move any limbs spontaneously?
- Does the patient have a tracheostomy in situ or portable ventilator? (This may give a clue as to the height of the lesion.)

History
- A history of trauma is common in the spinally injured patient.
- Ask how long ago the injury occurred, and for how long the patient was initially hospitalised.
- Ask about initial treatment, including surgery.
- Patients are often very knowledgeable about the level of their lesion and the associated sensorimotor deficits.
- Did the injury result in complete spinal cord transection?
- For thoracic lesions and above, ask about autonomic symptoms triggered by everyday activities, surgery, and other events.
- Ask about chronic complications from the injury:
  - chronic pain
  - skeletal muscle spasms
  - pressure area care problems
  - pulmonary and urinary tract infections
  - thermoregulatory disorders
  - anaemia.
- What limitations does the level of injury place on the patient's lifestyle, and how have they adapted to this?
- Obtain details of previous surgery and anaesthetics, and whether there were any associated problems.
- Obtain a list of current medications and any allergies which may be present (e.g. latex).

Physical examination
- You should attempt to correlate physical signs with the level of the injury.
- Remember that there will be lower motor neurone signs at the level of the lesion:
  - weakness
  - wasting
  - loss of tone
  - reduced reflexes
  - fasciculation.
- There will be upper motor neurone signs below the level of the lesion:
  - paralysis, wasting
  - increased tone and clonus
  - hyperreflexia
  - extensor plantar response.
- There will be complete sensory loss below the level of the lesion.
- Bradycardia and heart block will usually not occur unless the lesion is above T4.
- Systematic examination is best carried out with the patient supine, and should include:
  - inspection for fasciculations and muscle wasting
  - test tone at knees, hips and ankles; test for clonus
  - test power in upper and lower limbs, if any present
  - test lower limb reflexes: knee jerk, ankle jerk, plantar reflex
  - determine sensory level, comparing left and right; time will probably preclude testing of multiple modalities (touch, pain, temperature, vibration and proprioception).
- If time permits, assess the patient's airway and listen to the praecordium and posterior chest.

Useful statements
'Mrs H is a young woman who sustained a mid-thoracic spinal injury in a diving accident 6 years ago, leaving her paraplegic with a loss of bladder and bowel function. Despite this, she maintains a rigorous lifestyle and has had no cardiac or respiratory compromise. Complications of the injury have included relapsing urinary tract infections, and two episodes of autonomic hyperreflexia associated with catheterisation. On examination there is paralysis and wasting of both lower limbs with significant muscle spasm, increased tone, hyperreflexia of knee and ankle jerks with clonus demonstrated at the right ankle on hyperextension. There is an extensor plantar response.

'There is sensory loss below T5 dermatomal level.'

Investigations
- Radiological investigation of the injury: X-rays, CT scan
- Spirometry
- ECG for high thoracic lesions
- Full blood count, urea and electrolytes
- Urine microscopy and culture.

Topics for discussion
- Pathophysiology of autonomic hyperreflexia: what factors increase the likelihood?
- Prevention and treatment of autonomic hyperreflexia
- Muscle relaxants in spinal injuries, acute and chronic
- Central neuraxial blockade for surgery
- Controversies in neuroprotection for acute spinal cord injury
- Airway management of the patient with a suspected cervical injury
- Controversies in radiological diagnosis of spinal injuries.

13. The patient with muscular dystrophy

Possible clinical scenario
Mr K A is a 19-year-old man with weakness. He is confined to a wheelchair. Please take a brief history and conduct a neurological examination of his upper limbs.

Appropriate thoughts
Some causes of weakness in a male patient of this age include muscular dystrophy, myasthenia (although unusual to be wheelchair-bound with treatment), myotonic dystrophy, cerebral palsy and motor neurone disease. (Of the muscular dystrophies, Becker has similar features to Duchenne, but is usually less severe, is of later onset, and is less progressive. Fascioscapulohumeral dystrophy is nearly as common as Duchenne, but less than 20% will require a wheelchair before the age of 40.)

First impressions
- Examination patients may be present with a carer, who can provide much useful history.
- There may be obvious muscle wasting.
- Is there kyphoscoliosis present?

- Patients with myotonic dystrophy have characteristic facies, baldness and visual problems.

History
- Patients should be able to give you a diagnosis.
- Ask about onset of symptoms, symptom progression and functional limitations.
- Does the patient have any cardiorespiratory problems?
- Are there any problems with speech, swallowing or oesophageal reflux?
- Have there been any recent anaesthetics, operations or intensive care admissions?
- Is anyone else in the family affected? (Sketching a brief family tree may give clues to the genetic inheritance, and hence diagnosis; be aware though that cases may be the result of spontaneous gene mutation.)

Physical examination
- Patients with muscular dystrophy usually have severe proximal weakness. Deep tendon reflexes tend to be preserved proportional to the amount of remaining muscle mass. Sensation is usually not affected.
- Further examination in consideration for surgery would include cardiovascular examination (patients often develop cardiomyopathy and may have mitral valve prolapse) and respiratory examination (pneumonia and respiratory failure are common terminal events).

Useful statements
'Mr A is a young man who suffers from Duchenne muscular dystrophy. He has been a recent inpatient with left-sided pneumonia, from which he has now recovered. His condition was diagnosed at the age of 3, and he has been wheelchair-bound since the age of 11. Progression seems to have been rapid in the last year, with worsening weakness, reduced functional mobility and increased frequency of respiratory infections. He has difficulty swallowing and has a PEG in situ. While he is still cared for by his parents at home, he is currently being considered for full-time nursing care in a palliative care centre.

'On examination there is severe muscle wasting of all muscle groups, and obvious kyphoscoliosis. There is marked weakness of all upper limb muscle groups, reduced grip strength, demonstrably present but reduced biceps, triceps and supinator reflexes, and no loss of sensation to light touch.'

Investigations
- Creatine kinase is always high in patients with Duchenne muscular dystrophy.
- Routine preoperative screening would include respiratory function testing, chest X-ray and ECG.
- Echocardiography may be extremely useful if surgery is planned.

Topics for discussion
- Genetic inheritance of the different muscular dystrophies
- Use of depolarising and non-depolarising relaxants, volatile agents, including dosage
- Pre-medication if surgery is planned
- What is your anaesthetic technique for this patient if appendicitis is suspected?

14. The patient with multiple sclerosis

Possible clinical scenario

Mrs O W is a 29-year-old woman who presented several years ago with transient right hemiparesis. Please take a history of her illness and examine her cranial nerves.

Appropriate thoughts

- The history suggests a central nervous system disorder, and the patient is too young to be suffering from an atherosclerotic cause (unless it was a severe familial hyperlipidaemia). Other possible causes include hemiplegic migraine, paradoxical emboli or multiple sclerosis.
- Focus on taking a thorough history and demonstrating a good cranial nerve examination technique until the nature of the problem becomes more obvious. Patients with multiple sclerosis are usually very well informed about their disease.

First impressions

- Between exacerbations some patients may appear completely well with near complete recovery of symptoms. Others may suffer a more progressive form of the disease without distinct episodes.

History

- Diagnosis of multiple sclerosis requires separate episodes of central nervous system events.
- Ask about onset and offset of symptoms, which may include limb paresis, parasthesiae, ataxia, vertigo, visual disturbance, seizures and pseudobulbar palsy.
- Ask if there are any precipitating factors for attacks (stress, extremes of temperature, intercurrent illnesses, exercise).
- Discuss how the illness impacts on functions of daily living.
- Ask about past and current treatments (which may include carbamazepine, steroids, interferon and some cytotoxics, and rarely plasmapheresis; baclofen and dantrolene may relieve muscle spasm).
- Urinary retention and urgency are common.

Physical examination

- Even with the constraints of the examination format there should be time to perform a thorough cranial nerve examination.
- Note that signs can be extremely variable; there may be loss of visual acuity with central/hemianopic field defects, internuclear ophthalmoplegia (weakness of adduction in one eye and nystagmus in the other), facial weakness and swallowing disorders. In general, cranial nerve signs occur less frequently than long tract signs.
- Further CNS examination may reveal sensory defects, especially to vibration, cerebellar signs (such as ataxia or intention tremor) and variable patterns of spastic motor weakness.

Useful statements

'Mrs W first presented 3 years ago with a sudden fall at home and weakness of her right arm and leg, which resolved after several days. Investigations for cerebrovascular disease were negative. Approximately 9 months ago she suffered an episode of dizziness, reduced co-ordination and difficulty maintaining her balance, and was admitted to hospital, at which point a diagnosis of multiple sclerosis was made. These symptoms also resolved after 2 weeks. Since that time she has also suffered from blurred and double vision, which is always present, but fluctuates in severity. She has no other functional limitations at present but has chosen to stop driving. She is currently taking 5 mg prednisone per day.

'On examination of her cranial nerves there are no visual field defects to gross testing. Eye movements are preserved, but there is sustained nystagmus in her right eye on rightward gaze, which may represent either internuclear ophthalmoplegia or cerebellar disease. Her tongue deviates to the right on protrusion, but there is no wasting or fasciculation. This may represent a right hypoglossal nerve lesion. There are no other obvious cranial nerve abnormalities.'

Investigations
- MRI is the imaging modality of choice and may show demyelinated plaques.
- CSF analysis may show leukocytosis, IgG bands and myelin basic protein.

Topics for discussion
- Autonomic instability and general anaesthesia
- Importance of temperature monitoring during anaesthesia
- Does general anaesthesia affect the course of the disease?
- Would you be prepared to administer an epidural in labour for this patient?

15. The patient with myasthenia gravis

Possible clinical scenario
Mrs U S, 35, has a history of difficulty swallowing and fatigue on exertion. Please take a history and examine her upper limbs, and other areas as you see fit.

Appropriate thoughts
- The given history suggests a neuromuscular problem.
- With myasthenia it is important to assess the severity of the illness, current treatment, and anticipate questions related to the conduct of anaesthesia in such a patient.

First impressions
- Limb girdle and bulbar involvement suggests more severe disease; a degree of ptosis may be evident, and the quality of the patient's voice may deteriorate after a few minutes; all of these may depend on the timing and effectiveness of current treatment.
- A characteristic myasthenic 'snarl' may be evident on smiling.

History
- Ask about duration and severity of symptoms, especially limb weakness and chewing or swallowing difficulty (which predict the need for intra- and postoperative airway protection).
- Ocular symptoms of ptosis and diplopia are common.
- Is there significant respiratory impairment?
- What functional limitations are present?

- Previous anaesthetic history is of great importance.
- What treatment has been undertaken? Thymectomy, immunosuppressives, immunoglobulin, plasmapheresis may have been tried. Symptomatic control is usually with pyridostigmine; daily dosage >700 mg is a predictor of the need for postoperative ventilation.

Physical examination

- Test for easy fatiguability of the upper limbs (holding above the head); power will be globally reduced.
- Reflexes in the upper limb should be preserved and there is no sensory loss.
- Ask the patient to keep gazing upward, which may reveal weakness of the eyelid and oculomotor muscles.

Useful statements

'Mrs S first reported symptoms of weakness and fatigue 4 years ago, and was unable to undertake her regular gym training sessions. A diagnosis of myasthenia gravis was made, and she has been on medical therapy since. Her limb weakness improved, but in the last few months has deteriorated. Diplopia became a more significant problem and she was unable to leave her house. Swallowing difficulties with solid food appeared at the same time, and she has had two urgent gastroscopies to retrieve food boluses since then. There have been no reported respiratory problems, but she does not walk further than 200 m due to fatigue. Her current dose of pyridostigmine is 600 mg per day, and her symptoms noticeably worsen after one missed dose. She is currently being investigated and worked up for thymoma removal.

'On examination, I noticed that her voice became husky after a few minutes speaking. She has obvious ptosis. Upper limb examination reveals easy muscle fatiguability, with overhead arm lift unable to be sustained for greater than 20 seconds. Grip strength is initially normal, but fades after about 10 seconds. Reflexes are normal and there is no sensory deficit to light touch.'

Investigations

- Diagnostic tests may include assay of antibodies against acetylcholine receptors, electromyography and edrophonium challenge.
- Investigations for thymoma will usually include chest X-ray and MRI scanning.
- Preoperatively spirometry is very useful; patients with markedly reduced vital capacity are more likely to require postoperative ventilatory support.

Topics for discussion

- How would you anaesthetise this patient for emergency laparotomy?
- Management of anticholinesterase therapy in the perioperative period
- Under what circumstances could the patient be extubated at the end of surgery?
- Differentiation of myasthenic crisis from cholinergic crisis.

16. The patient with chronic renal impairment

Possible clinical scenario

Mrs E N, 49, presents because of a blocked A-V fistula. Please take a history and examine as you see fit.

Appropriate thoughts
- You should have guessed by now that the patient is likely to have renal failure.
- It is important to elucidate the cause, any complications and current treatment.

First impressions
- Is the patient an inpatient? Is there a vascath or peritoneal dialysis device in situ?
- You may gain an impression of the patient's overall hydration state.

History
- Ask when renal failure was diagnosed and what led to the diagnosis. Does the patient know the underlying cause for renal disease?
  - glomerulonephritis (primary, or as part of another disease, e.g. lupus)
  - analgesic nephropathy
  - diabetic nephropathy
  - hypertensive nephrosclerosis
  - ureteric reflux
  - polycystic kidney disease.
- Ask about progression of the disease and its treatment, including fluid restriction, dialysis (peritoneal and haemodialysis), transplantation (previous or pending) and other medical treatments (e.g. for hypertension).
- Have there been any major complications of the disease or its treatment?
  - hypertension, anaemia, uraemia, cardiac failure, gout, acute fluid overload
  - dialysis access problems, blocked or infected shunts, peritonitis
  - transplant problems: rejection, infection, complications of immunosuppression.
- Discuss functional limitations on the patient's activity, and how the dialysis impacts on their life.
- Ask about concomitant medical conditions, medications, problems with previous surgery and anaesthesia and allergies.

Physical examination
- Make an assessment of the hydration of the patient. Is she clinically anaemic?
- Measure the blood pressure, and ask for the patient's ideal body weight.
- Examine any dialysis access points, including fistulae for patency, thrombosis or infection, indwelling central venous access lines and peritoneal access points.
- Examine the chest and listen for a pericardial rub or evidence of cardiac failure. Listen to the lung fields.
- Examine the abdomen for scars of previous surgery (dialysis, transplants). Palpate for organomegaly and ascites.
- Examine the legs for oedema, bruising and peripheral neuropathy.

Useful statements
'Mrs N has a 12-year history of chronic renal impairment caused by membranous glomerulonephritis for which she has been receiving intermittent haemodialysis three times a week for 6 years via an arteriovenous fistula fashioned on her left wrist. Prior to that she had received peritoneal dialysis, which was discontinued due to several serious peritoneal infections. Four days ago it was noted that her A-V fistula was completely thrombosed. She is currently an inpatient receiving haemodialysis via a vascath placed in her right subclavian vein, pending new A-V fistula formation tomorrow. She leads an active lifestyle despite her illness. She is

not on the waiting list for a renal transplant because of her own personal cultural beliefs. On examination she is normotensive and her hydration appears normal, consistent with her dialysis last night.'

Investigations
- Urea, creatinine and serum electrolytes, creatinine clearance and plasma creatinine/urea ratio
- Chest X-ray – look for acute pericarditis, position of vascath
- Full blood count
- ECG
- ABG – look for metabolic acidosis.

Topics for discussion
- Timing of dialysis and elective surgery, perioperative fluid management
- Complications and mortality from dialysis
- Electrolyte disturbances and their emergency treatment
- Anaesthetic techniques for A-V fistula formation: general versus regional
- Management of coagulation problems in renal failure
- Pharmacology of anaesthetic agents in renal failure.

17. The patient with chronic liver disease

Possible clinical scenario
Mr E X, aged 63, has been feeling unwell for many weeks. Please take a history and conduct an abdominal examination.

Appropriate thoughts
The directed examination suggests the possibility of abdominal organomegaly.

First impressions
- Is the patient jaundiced?
- Is the patient malnourished?
- Other immediate clues to chronic liver disease may include tattoos (a source of viral infection) or pigmentation (haemochromatosis).

History
- Ask the patient if they know the nature of their underlying condition. A diagnosis of cirrhosis is commonly caused by either chronic alcohol abuse or viral infection, although the differential diagnosis is large.
- What caused the patient to seek treatment? Common presenting complaints include:
  - weakness and fatigue
  - jaundice
  - abdominal pain or swelling (ascites)
  - altered mental state
  - pruritis.
- Ask about the duration of liver disease, including the following:
  - alcohol intake
  - intravenous drug addiction, tattoos, blood transfusions

 – overseas travel
 – drugs, e.g. isoniazid.
- Have there been any complications?
 – haematemesis from bleeding varices, melaena
 – ascites
 – encephalopathy
 – cholecystitis
 – pancreatitis.
- What treatment has the patient received (including investigations)?
 – liver biopsy
 – ascitic tap
 – protein and fluid restriction
 – gastroscopy and injection of varices, portocaval shunt.
- Enquire about restrictions on activity, and social impact of the disease.

Physical examination

You may be again directed by the examiner to start examination at the abdomen. The patient should be lying supine, with one pillow.
- As you approach the abdomen, you may notice other stigmata of chronic liver disease:
 – palmar erythema
 – bruising
 – spider naevi
 – yellow sclerae
 – fetor
 – gynaecomastia.
- Inspect the abdomen:
 – masses
 – distension
 – bruising
 – scars.
- Palpate all four quadrants:
 – hepatomegaly: massive, firm, tender, irregular, pulsatile
 – splenomegaly (consider rolling patient onto right side as well)
 – kidneys.
- Percuss:
 – approximate liver span
 – ascites: roll and test for shifting dullness.
- Auscultation:
 – bruits
 – friction rubs
 – presence of bowel sounds.
- Assess for the presence of hepatic encephalopathy:
 – asterixis/flap
 – constructional apraxia.

Useful statements

'Mr X is currently an inpatient and gives his presenting problem as cirrhosis. He is a vague historian. On further questioning he reports excessive alcohol consumption of at least 2 bottles of port per night over a period of approximately 40 years, which is the likely cause of his disease. He has undergone recent gastroscopy for haematemesis. He is unaware of any current medical treatments. On examination he is malnourished with several stigmata of chronic liver disease, including scleral jaundice, many spider naevi on his arms and trunk, palmar erythema and many large bruises. Examination of his abdomen reveals generalised distension. Both liver and spleen were palpable and both were significantly enlarged. I suspect the presence of ascites as evidenced by shifting dullness to percussion. The most likely diagnosis in this gentleman is cirrhosis caused by alcoholic hepatitis, and complicated by portal hypertension.'

Investigations
- Full blood count
- Urea and electrolytes, serum ammonia
- Transaminases, bilirubin, albumin, blood glucose
- Coagulation studies
- Ascitic fluid cytology, microscopy, culture and biochemistry
- Liver biopsy.

Topics for discussion
- Anaesthetic implications of chronic liver disease
- Child–Pugh classification of severity of liver disease
- Indications/contraindications for liver transplantation
- Differential diagnosis of hepatosplenomegaly
- Causes of acute hepatitis
- Risks of needle stick injury for hepatitis viruses
- Anaesthetic implications of chronic alcoholism.

18. The patient with an organ transplant

Possible clinical scenario
Mrs Q F, 36, presents for routine check-up after major surgery. Please take a history and examine her cardiovascular system.

Appropriate thoughts
There are few clues to go on here, unless the major surgery was on her cardiovascular system …

First impressions
- Unless major complications have intervened, the majority of patients with a solid organ transplant regain the function of the previously diseased organ.
- It is likely that the patient will appear fit and well, but this may depend on how long ago the operation took place. The patient may appear Cushingoid from steroid therapy.

History
- Most patients will be very well informed about the nature of their previous disease and treatment, and the diagnosis will quickly become obvious.
- Ask about the cause of previous cardiac failure (in this age group usually due to cardiomyopathy) and symptoms the patient was experiencing prior to surgery, including functional limitation and exercise tolerance.

- Ask about the patient's surgery: when and where, and whether there were any complications (the most common of these are rejection and infection). Coronary vascular disease and malignancy may be problems in later years, as may hyperlipidaemia and hypertension.
- Determine the patient's current exercise tolerance and functional reserve.
- Are they able to work?
- Ask about current medications, especially anti-hypertensives, cholesterol-lowering medication and immunosuppressants – have there been any adverse reactions from these?
- Ask about routine check-ups, including cardiac catheterisation and biopsies.
- Ask about any other co-existent diseases, previous anaesthetic problems and allergies.

Physical examination
- Perform your usual cardiovascular examination.
- Ask for the patient's weight and blood pressure.
- The transplanted heart lacks parasympathetic innervation, the resting heart rate is usually around 90 beats per minute, and sinus arrhythmia is lost.
- A small percentage of patients require a permanent pacemaker because of postoperative bradycardias.
- A median sternotomy scar will be present, as may scars over the right internal jugular vein (from endocardial biopsies).
- Listen for normal heart sounds and clear lung fields.

Useful statements
'Mrs F presents for routine cardiac catheterisation 3 years after successful heart transplantation. She suffered from severe cardiomyopathy prior to this, with rapid deterioration in functional status over 2 years. At the time of her operation she was bed-bound, suffered from severe orthopnoea and had an exercise tolerance of 10 metres on the flat. The operation proceeded uneventfully and there were no immediate postoperative complications. She has suffered some basal cell carcinomas on her skin since the operation, but few other problems with immunosuppression. She is working full-time and can walk for several kilometres a day.'

Investigations
- ECG: look for a second P wave (native + donor atrium; usually disappears), RBBB common
- Cardiac catheterisation data
- Echocardiography: look for intramural thrombi, ventricular function
- Full blood count and serum electrolytes
- Chest X-ray.

Topics for discussion
- Management of anaesthesia for elective surgery
- Infection prophylaxis
- Detection of postoperative ischaemia
- What signs and symptoms might alert you to the possibility of rejection?
- Long-term prognosis for transplant recipients.

Note that many candidates will sit the clinical examination in a major or capital city where transplant candidates (pre- and post-surgery) are readily available for participation in the medical vivas. The information presented above can be used in a first principles extrapolation for lung, kidney and liver transplants, i.e. cause and consequences of previous organ dysfunction, perioperative management and complications (including complications of immunosuppression), post-transplant function. You should be able to assess these patients as though they were appearing on your list for elective surgery, even if you are from a centre where transplant patients are a rarity.

19. The patient with rheumatoid arthritis

Possible clinical scenario
Mrs S A, aged 49, presents for metacarpophalangeal joint replacement of her hands. Please take a history and conduct a relevant examination.

Appropriate thoughts
- The operation should alert you to a possible diagnosis.
- Think of the articular and extra-articular manifestations of rheumatoid arthritis that may be of relevance to anaesthesia.

First impressions
- A diagnosis of rheumatoid arthritis may be obvious on first inspection.
- Does the patient look Cushingoid from steroid use?

History
- Determine if rheumatoid arthritis is the patient's main medical problem.
- Ask when the diagnosis was made and what symptoms, initially led to the diagnosis.
- Disease progression is important. Ask which joints are mainly affected, and specifically ask about the neck and jaw.
- Ask specifically about upper limb neurological symptoms, which may indicate nerve or spinal cord compression.
- Is the disease currently active? What functional impairment is present and in which joints? How does this impact on activities of daily living?
- Ask about past and present drug treatment.
- Have there been any problems related to pharmacological therapy?
- Obtain a list of all medications.
- Ask about previous anaesthetic problems and document any allergies.
- Remember non-articular symptoms of the disease:
  - dry or inflamed eyes
  - Raynaud's phenomenon
  - peripheral neuropathy
  - dyspnoea from anaemia or pleural effusion/fibrosis
  - chest pain typical of pericarditis
  - renal problems.

Physical examination
It may be useful to describe the articular changes seen in rheumatoid arthritis to the examiners as you find them.

- Upper limbs:
  - swan-neck and boutonnière deformities of the fingers
  - Z deformity of the thumb
  - ulnar deviation and palmar subluxation at the wrist
  - vasculitis may be evident in the nail-beds
  - look for muscle wasting on the palmar surface of the hands
  - evidence of previous surgery
  - rheumatoid nodules, if present.
- Feel and move any affected joints for swelling and range of movement and tenderness (be gentle).
- Test the patient's grip strength and hand function (ask the patient to undo and redo a button).
- Head and neck:
  - Look at the patient's posture and test the range of movement of the neck in all planes
  - Look for temporomandibular joint involvement (swelling and tenderness to palpation, clicking and grating with jaw opening)
  - Examine the eyes for redness and dryness and nodular scleritis
  - Listen for hoarseness, which may indicate cricoarytenoid involvement.
- Chest:
  - Listen to the heart for murmurs and pericardial rub
  - Listen to lung fields for signs of effusion or crepitations due to pulmonary fibrosis.
- Abdomen:
  - Look for splenomegaly if time permits (in Felty's syndrome, associated with neutropenia).

Investigations

- Serology: note that rheumatoid factor is neither particularly specific nor sensitive; urea and electrolytes for renal function
- X-rays of affected joints: look for joint erosion, destruction and swelling
- C-spine X-ray: when examining flexion and extension films look for atlanto-axial subluxation (seen as separation of anterior margin of odontoid process from posterior margin anterior arch of atlas >3–4 mm). If separation is severe, the odontoid process may protrude into foramen magnum and put pressure on spinal cord or impair blood flow through vertebral arteries. The odontoid may be eroded. Subluxation of other cervical vertebrae may occur.
- Echocardiography: look for pericardial effusion
- ECG: look for acute pericarditis, conduction defects from nodules
- Chest X-ray: look for thoracic manifestations of the disease
- FBC: check for anaemia, thrombocytopaenia
- Spirometry: look for a restrictive lung defect.

Useful statements

'Mrs A presents for her third metacarpophalangeal joint replacement operation. She has had rheumatoid arthritis for 15 years, and manifests severe changes of a symmetric polyarthropathy to the joints in her hands and wrists, which severely limit her functional activity. She has had no problems with her cervical spine or temporomandibular joint and to date no complications of her eyes, lungs, heart or kidneys. Her current medications include aspirin, prednisolone and methotrexate, which are only partially effective in relieving her symptoms. Examination of her neck and airway is unremarkable.'

Topics for discussion
- Diagnosis of cervical spine, temporomandibular joint, laryngeal involvement
- Complications of pharmacological therapy: aspirin, NSAID, steroids, methotrexate, penicillamine, gold, azathioprine, cyclosporin
- Perioperative glucocorticoid supplementation
- Airway management for distal limb surgery
- Extra-articular manifestations of the disease
- Intraoperative positioning and monitoring difficulties.

20. The patient with ankylosing spondylitis

Possible clinical scenario
Mr L O, 29, requires insertion of lower jaw prosthetic dental implants under general anaesthesia. He has a long history of back and hip pain. Please take a brief history and examine his airway and axial skeleton.

Appropriate thoughts
- The given history suggests orthopaedic injury or arthritides. The examination request raises the possibility of spondylitis.
- Perhaps the impending surgery is for dental trauma from difficult intubation?

First impressions
- Ankylosis of the spine may lead to an unusually stiff posture.
- Kyphosis may be obvious.

History
- Taking a brief dental history may be appropriate in this case.
- Ask about onset, severity and progression of back and hip pain. Patients usually complain of back pain radiating to the sacro-iliac joints and hips, which is worse at night and improves after movement.
- Tendon and ligament inflammation is common, especially Tendoachilles, costochondritis.
- Ask about visual symptoms – uveitis/iritis is common and may be severe.
- Ask about cardiovascular and renal disease; there are associations with aortitis, aortic regurgitation, pulmonary fibrosis and amyloid deposits.
- Ask about previous anaesthetic or airway difficulties.
- Specific problems include temporomandibular joint dysfunction, cervical fusion, atlanto-axial subluxation, risk of occult cervical fracture with minimal trauma, cricoarytenoid arthritis; neuraxial block may be impossible (paramedian spinal may be best option); patient positioning may be difficult; limited chest expansion may be present.
- Ask about functional limitations and current treatment.

Physical examination
- Care should be spent assessing the airway for features listed above.
- Observe any kyphosis of the spine and assess degree of movement of all parts of the spine.

- Feel for specific tenderness in the spine and sacro-iliac joints; assess hip range of motion.
- Examine the chest (thoracic expansion specifically) and auscultate the heart and lungs.

Useful statements

'Mr O is a young man who suffered dental trauma from a difficult intubation while undergoing appendicectomy 7 months ago. He carries a letter and Medic Alert bracelet detailing this; the main problems seem to have been with jaw opening and limited neck movement. He was diagnosed with ankylosing spondylitis as a teenager, which affects his entire spine and his sacro-iliac joints. He has no history of cardiac disease, but suffers from uveitis. On examination there is fixed kyphosis of the thoracic spine and loss of lumbar lordosis. There is markedly reduced neck flexion and extension with some preservation of rotation. There is tenderness over both sacro-iliac joints and reduced hip flexion. My main concern is airway management for the impending surgery.'

Investigations

- Preoperative respiratory function testing and echocardiography may be indicated if evidence of extra-articular disease is present.
- Neck and spine X-rays will outline extent of disease.
- FBE may show normochromic anaemia.

Topics for discussion

- Technique of intubation
- What do you do if awake fibre-optic intubation fails?
- The patient returns 1 year later for repair of ruptured Achilles tendon. What other problems do you anticipate?

21. The patient with trisomy 21

Possible clinical scenario

Mr T O is 24 and due to undergo dental examination under anaesthesia. He is present with a carer. Please take a history and conduct a brief examination.

Appropriate thoughts

- Patients with Trisomy 21 (Down Syndrome) will occasionally appear in the medical vivas. They will often be present with a relative or carer, who may provide the bulk of relevant history. It is important to have a gentle, kind approach.
- You should be considering systemic manifestations of the condition.

First impressions

The diagnosis can be made from the characteristic facies.

History

While many patients with Trisomy 21 have intellectual impairment, there is a wide variation in cognitive abilities in this group of patients. You may be asked to direct your questions to the carer present.

- Ask about complications and associations of the syndrome that have been encountered in the past:
  - congenital heart disease (especially endocardial cushion defects/VSD/patent ductus/tetralogy of Fallot), corrective surgery, cyanotic episodes, pulmonary hypertension
  - eye problems: strabismus, cataracts
  - hypothyroidism
  - central or obstructive sleep apnoea, susceptibility to respiratory infection
  - joint problems, including cervical instability
  - epilepsy
  - hearing problems
  - immunosuppression and increased risk of malignancy, e.g. leukaemia.
- Ask about the patient's current level of functioning at home and in the community.
- Ask about previous operations and anaesthetics and any problems encountered.
- Obtain a list of medications and ask about any allergies.

Physical examination
- Some time should be spent focusing on aspects of the patient's airway. Particular problems include:
  - macroglossia
  - micrognathia
  - short, broad neck
  - atlanto-axial instability in about 15% of patients: usually asymptomatic
  - subglottic stenosis less common in adults
  - generalised joint laxity, including temporomandibular joint
  - high arched palate.
- Examine the cardiovascular system, in particular looking for evidence of previous surgery and any cardiac murmurs that may be present.
- Look for evidence of pulmonary hypertension or right ventricular hypertrophy.

Useful statements
'Mr O is a young man born with Trisomy 21. He has a history of a small ventricular septal defect, which has required no further treatment. Other manifestations of the condition include epilepsy, which is currently well controlled on sodium valproate, and moderate intellectual impairment. There has been no problem with operations or anaesthesia in the past. On examination, many characteristic features of Trisomy 21 are present. My concerns relating to management of his airway include macroglossia and micrognathia with reduced neck movement in all directions. Cardiac auscultation reveals a loud pansystolic murmur throughout the praecordium consistent with a ventricular septal defect. I would seek further information before embarking on the proposed surgery.'

Investigations
- Previous anaesthetic records may provide much useful information
- Echocardiography
- ECG
- Thyroid function tests
- Cervical spine X-rays.

Topics for discussion
- Aetiology of the disorder
- Treatment of hypoxia/right to left shunting in children
- Approach to airway management in this patient
- Should cervical spine X-rays be routine in all Down syndrome patients?

Chapter 5

The anaesthesia vivas

There is no squabbling so violent as that between people who accepted an idea yesterday and those who will accept the same idea tomorrow.
CHRISTOPHER MORLEY

Overview

The anaesthesia vivas are a searching component of the examination: in eight short interviews the examiners try to ascertain the depth and breadth of candidates' knowledge, and whether they have met the standard to work as a junior consultant anaesthetist. This section has the greatest proportion of marks attached to it (48%) and is also the only part of the FANZCA examination that it is obligatory to pass in order to pass the examination. (As mentioned previously, you also need to pass any one of the other three parts, and get at least 50% overall.)

The examiners assess clinical judgement, prioritisation, interpretation of complex situations, anticipation of clinical actions and their sequelae, the application of clinical experience with the knowledge of potential pitfalls and an ability to 'think on one's feet'.

Performance strategies

If you are travelling to the anaesthesia viva examination from interstate or overseas, make sure you plan your flight and accommodation well in advance. The college website has information to assist you in this regard. It is best to fly to the host city at least one day before the exam to give you time to settle in and determine your route to the venue. Again, try and minimise the amount of reading or study you do the day before the exam.

When choosing accommodation it may be worth liaising with other colleagues who are sitting the examination, as you may get a discount for a group booking. Make sure you stay somewhere comfortable that has room service, as you may not feel like dining out. Both Sydney and Melbourne have large, good quality, reasonably priced hotels within walking distance of the examination venues. Talk to senior colleagues to gain advice on preferred places to stay. Whether you take your family with you is a personal choice – some enjoy solitude, whereas others prefer the distraction of company.

Get as much sleep as you can, eat as well as you can and allow plenty of preparation time on the day of the examination. Unpack your clothes the day before and make sure you have everything you need. This gives you time to buy any item you may have forgotten (such as a shirt).

When dressing for the examination it is important to create a good impression. This normally implies a long-sleeved shirt, suit and tie for men, and similarly professional attire for women. Try and find shoes that are comfortable, as you will be spending a long time in them. Daring costumes and colourful outfits are generally not appropriate.

Arrive at the examination venue in plenty of time, and use whatever strategies you can to calm your nerves. You will inevitably be more anxious than at the written exam because you are in a foreign environment with unfamiliar faces, and your performance is under greater scrutiny with less anonymity. Performance anxiety can be an overwhelming entity for some candidates. The best strategies to combat this include effective preparation and exhaustive practice leading up to the exam. Counselling and professional psychological training can aid the performance of those candidates who are severely affected.

At the rest station avoid the temptation to dissect previous vivas with other candidates (some of whom will be excessively keen to do so). If refreshments are provided, partake of them frugally, especially caffeinated drinks early on in the rotation when your bladder may be at its most irritable.

The viva

All candidates in a four viva rotation are presented with the same clinical scenario and the same initial question, and the theme of the viva and its key issues are the same for each candidate. The examiners will have agreed on a marking guide in advance, and the areas to be emphasised. However, the examiners are given scope to explore the level of understanding within this framework, and so they may ask additional questions to achieve this. They have a list of supplementary questions for the end of the viva in case a candidate moves through the material quickly. For these reasons each candidate will not be asked exactly the same questions as their colleagues.

The anaesthesia viva is unlikely to ask for purely factual knowledge or the recall of a cognitive model, as such abilities are better tested in the multiple choice or short answer papers. Candidates are expected to describe the management of situations as they would in real life.

The 15 minutes of the viva will pass surprisingly quickly. Candidates will usually be addressed by one examiner, who will be seated directly opposite with the viva outline and a marking book. These are usually partly obscured by the name plate that sits on the desk of the examiner, thereby denying those candidates with the peculiar ability to read upside-down an unfair advantage. As you give appropriate responses you may notice some of the examiners ticking the marking sheet, which can be reassuring. However, many of the examiners may make few notes or ticks during the viva, and complete the entire marking process after the candidate has left the room. Do not panic if there is minimal 'tick action' during the course of the viva.

There may be an observer in the room, who will normally position themselves beside the other examiner. They will be introduced at the beginning of the viva, but will not say anything from that point on. Look at the examiner asking the questions and ignore the observer. The observer may be a junior examiner observing a more senior colleague, or a senior examiner observing another examiner to assess their technique. All examiners expect to be observed at least once during an examination, and this process, instituted by the college, provides a form of quality control.

The tone you should adopt during the vivas is that of a respectful but competent colleague. If you are an authority on a particular topic this will soon become obvious to the examiner from the answers you give to the questions posed. If you have never been exposed to the particular scenario in question this will also usually be obvious to the examiners. It is not appropriate to refuse to answer a question based on the fact that you have not previously been exposed to that situation. It is not possible for marks to be awarded on the basis of no response. It is better to say: 'While I have never performed this technique/seen this condition/caused this complication personally, the most appropriate course of action I would consider in that circumstance would be …'

Similarly, if you envisage a viva following a particular path (e.g. you suspect your choice of general anaesthesia may result in failed tracheal intubation) you cannot refuse to carry out a certain action if it is reasonable for normal anaesthetic practice. It wastes time to argue the point with the examiners, and they will eventually take you where they want you to go anyway. Remember the viva is reasonably structured and agreed upon among the examiners beforehand, so the script will be more or less followed. It is wise not to 'second guess' the topics that will be covered in a viva from the opening statement presented, as they often cover many areas that are unrelated. Generally there will be three major themes in the viva. You must be nimble of mind to rapidly adapt to the changing circumstances presented.

It is also unwise to predict what major areas you will be examined in. While it is likely there will be a major question each on obstetrics, paediatrics, chronic pain, neuroanaesthesia, vascular anaesthesia, difficult airway management, ambulatory anaesthesia and medicolegal/welfare issues, more than one of these areas can easily be accommodated in a single viva. Likewise, the major areas may occupy vivas in the examination sessions held on the other day by the other group of candidates (so you may, for example, sit an exam with no questions on obstetrics or paediatrics at all).

The management of crisis situations is also likely to crop up in many of the scenarios. Simple statements such as: 'I would handle that using the COVER algorithm' or 'I would apply ATLS guidelines' are unlikely to impress the examiners unless you elaborate further. The examiners want to know what you will actually do, so tell them. It is the verbalisation of your actions that lets them know you will handle a crisis appropriately and therefore deserve the marks. If there seems to be an obvious solution to a critical incident problem, state this at the beginning along with the appropriate treatment.

There has been less focus on anatomy in the anaesthesia vivas in recent years. Anatomy questions lend themselves to being assessed in the written components of the exam, which is more suited to the examination of pure factual knowledge. However, an understanding of applied anatomy relating to areas such as regional blocks or vascular access would be expected and may be incorporated into part of the viva. Similar observations can be made on the assessment of a candidate's knowledge of anaesthetic equipment. While the days of the examiner whipping out a skull or some treasured old piece of junk midway through a viva are unlikely to return, it is unwise to gamble and completely ignore the study of these areas.

You are also reminded that investigations will be presented to you in association with many of the anaesthesia viva scenarios, and not just saved for the medical vivas. This is more likely than in the past, as there is no longer a dedicated investigation viva to specifically examine this area.

The examiners realise that the examination is a very stressful situation for you. They appreciate that under such circumstances some people may freeze up or not perform at their best. Poor performance in one viva may adversely affect your performance in the next viva if you dwell on it rather than concentrating on the issue at hand. This may occur even if you have expert knowledge in that particular area. However, performance under pressure is also part of your daily work and some degree of cool-headedness in a stressful situation is to be expected, whether or not the handling of exam and work stress are closely related. At all times listen carefully to what is asked. Answer what is asked, rather than sprouting what you know. Each desk in the examination venue has a ready supply of water and tissues should you require them.

Should you say something 'outrageous' (usually due to a slip of the tongue or an honest mistake), or embark on a plan that is not within mainstream anaesthetic thinking, the examiner will usually try to give you a chance to retract your words. Words from the examiner, such as 'Sorry, can you repeat that?' or 'Is that really what you would do?', should not be looked upon as a challenge to stand by the courage of your convictions. Continuing to stick with a dangerous course of action following the opportunity for redemption is likely to lead to failure of the viva. Politely ask the examiner to repeat the previous question, then think carefully about the answer you gave. If it was patently absurd (e.g. 'I would give 100 mg of adrenaline'), then simply apologise and give a more appropriate answer. If you suddenly have insight where you did not before, then say something like 'On reflection, my preferred course of action would be ...' . The viva can then continue on a more favourable course.

In general, the examiners will try to structure the questions in such a way that you are not put in the position of producing a list. However, if the examiner asks for a list of possibilities, enumerate these as logically as you can. The same list given in a structured way will score better than a randomly assembled group of facts. If the examiner then asks: 'Is there anything else?', sometimes with the pen poised over their notes, it is likely you have forgotten something important and you are being given the opportunity to score more points.

Remember that the focus of the examination is for you prove to the college that you are knowledgeable and safe to work as a specialist anaesthetist. It is perfectly reasonable to say what you normally do in a particular situation, or to outline a course of action based on your experience, but if that course of action is revolutionary, non-mainstream, experimental or simply dangerous, you are probably better to keep it to yourself (and seriously consider changing your practice). It is worth keeping in mind that each viva is jointly prepared by a number of examiners, and therefore the expected responses will represent a consensus of mainstream thinking.

Do not enter the viva examination with the expectation that all examiners will be reassuring, friendly, smiling and gentle, as this is unlikely to be the case. Some examiners will go out of their way to put you at ease, but others may take a more formal, interrogative approach. Many of the examiners also take the approach of trying not to let their mannerisms, comments or tone of voice reflect how well you are doing. A seriously unemotional deadpan approach can be unsettling, but just ignore it. It is an attempt to try to be consistent across the range of candidates. Do not feel intimidated or discriminated against if you receive (in your opinion) a particularly brutal group of examiners. The marking system is as fair as possible and under constant review, so there is actually very little room for the personality of the examiner to play a part in the marks you receive for your answers.

Many candidates focus on mnemonics and prepared answers for introductory statements. For example, when asked how to give an anaesthetic for a particular surgery, a typical statement might go something like this: 'Having performed my usual preoperative assessment of the patient, including appropriate history, physical examination and review of relevant investigation results, and having organised appropriate consent and premedication of the patient, I would check my anaesthetic machine and ancillary equipment, ensure the availability of an appropriate anaesthetic assistant, and draw up and label the drugs I would use.' Then it is possible to launch into specific concerns for the case in question, including an appreciation of potential complications and pitfalls.

The advantage of this approach is that it takes only 20 seconds to regurgitate and covers a wealth of important information, showing how safe you are. Without such a system candidates often fumble around all of the above points, make significant errors of omission and waste a lot of time. However, you should make sure your statements are appropriate to the given situation. Be aware that such an approach may become tiresome for the examiners to listen to a hundred times, and they may fast-forward you through your spiel and ask you a more specific question. Note that at any stage they may interrupt you and ask for more detail ('What history do you normally take?' 'How would you assess your anaesthetic machine for leaks upstream of the common gas outlet?'). Also note that such an opening approach may not answer the specific question posed. If the opening question asks for specific investigations for a certain medical condition, then answer that directly. Many of the questions will be designed to ask a very specific question so as to avoid such rote introductions. You must be quick on your toes and flexible to the situation. The best way to achieve this is with practice.

Other useful statements during the vivas should be used to convey your appreciation of the urgency of a situation: 'This is an emergency' or 'This is a critical situation' or 'I would immediately hit the arrest alarm and call for help'. Once again, such statements need to be appropriate to the situation. Such bravado in response to mild laryngospasm or a blood pressure of 90 mmHg systolic is a gross overreaction and will not impress the examiners.

Viva technique is extremely important, and can only be achieved through practice. Practice within your study group is convenient and useful, and may bolster your speaking confidence. Be wary of remaining entirely within this comfort zone, however. Practise with as many different senior colleagues as possible, including those with whom you do not feel at ease. Ask for an appraisal of your technique, not just your knowledge.

Make a conscious effort to sit up straight and try to keep your hands still. Speak slowly and clearly. In the stress of the situation, many candidates rush their answers and talk incredibly quickly, omitting critical information in the process. When asked a question, force yourself to pause for a couple of seconds and consider the question carefully. Try not to 'um' and 'ah'. Sound confident, but not arrogant. While it may brighten the examiners' day if you smile occasionally, humour and one-liners are generally not appropriate in the exam. Even the best amateur comedian is unlikely to impress if, during a cardiac arrest scenario, he calls for help and a change of underwear.

Anaesthesia viva topics

It is impossible to cover, in any great detail, all the topics that could reasonably be asked in the anaesthesia vivas.

The following list comprises major topics that have been asked in the last 5 years (2005–09). Each question is followed by the sitting number (1 or 2) and year of origin.

This list may be used as a source of questions for practising viva technique, as well as helping prepare for the written examination. The previous examination reports (which are the source for the list that follows) are a very good guide to the type of questions that will be asked, and should be looked over carefully. The information provided in these has become much more detailed in the last couple of years.

While this list is large, most subjects will be covered during 4 years of anaesthetic training and preparation for the multiple choice question examination. It is worth noting which specific questions have been asked in the previous four or five examinations and reading the examiners' report on topics that have been answered poorly – these topics are a good source of future exam questions. Some questions are 'classics' and will keep being repeated due to their nature and clinical problems they pose, e.g. myasthenia gravis, perioperative anticoagulation and fractured neck of femur.

You should also consider how two or three topics could be combined in one scenario, e.g. aortic stenosis in a patient with an intracranial aneurysm for a coiling procedure at a remote location.

The other good source for revision topics are the college curriculum module document and part C of the college learning portfolio (clinical skills, drills and procedures). Between them these provide a good checklist of the knowledge, skills, attitudes and behaviours that the college considers important in a consultant anaesthetist. Any of these should be considered fair game to produce an anaesthesia viva topic.

If you can glance through these various lists and are confident of giving an expert dissertation on all the topics you are probably in very good shape for the anaesthesia viva examination. Consider potential controversies that may arise in a discussion of each of the following. The examiners will want you to be aware of potential pitfalls of any course of action you advocate.

Please note that many of the following viva topics involve a number of themes and cover several subject areas.

Airway

- Plan the airway management of uncooperative, developmentally delayed 20-year-old with a grade 4 Mallampati view for restorative dental work. (2/09)
- Form a plan for airway management in a patient with retrosternal thyroid and significant airway obstruction. (2/09)
- Assess and manage a difficult airway (food bolus in oesophagus). (1/09)
- Manage accidental intraoperative removal of airway by the surgeon. (1/09)
- Management of the obstructed endotracheal tube in tonsillectomy. (2/08)
- Management of post-extubation laryngospasm. (2/08)
- Management of the dislodged endotracheal tube intraoperatively. (2/08)
- Management of gas induction for an autistic 17-year-old with dental abscess. (1/08)

- Airway options for the obese 35-year-old with severe stridor presenting to the emergency department. (1/08)
- Airway management of 39-year-old intellectually impaired woman with large goitre. (2/07)
- Gas induction in an obese adult using a circle system and then placement of laryngeal mask, showing knowledge of the relationship between flow rates and changing gas concentrations. (1/07)
- Outline a plan for evaluating and securing the airway in a patient with potential tracheal injury, including the place of fibre-optic or rigid bronchoscopy. (1/07)
- Airway assessment and intubation technique for a patient with cervical canal stenosis. (1/07)
- Describe how you would teach rapid sequence induction, and safely manage failed intubation. (2/06)
- Evaluation of the airway in a 65-year-old man added acutely to your list for biopsy of a right-sided supraglottic carcinoma. (1/06)
- Immediate management of trail-bike rider with stridor, blood-stained saliva and sitting forward who has a neck injury following collision with a wire fence. (1/06)
- Airway management in patient with a penetrating eye injury sustained 7 hours ago while eating lunch. (2/05)

Blood transfusion/coagulation
- Diagnose (and interpret appropriate lab results) and manage severe intraoperative coagulopathy in multitrauma patient. (2/09)
- Diagnose and manage transfusion-related acute lung injury (including ABG interpretation). (2/09)
- Interpret coagulation screen and manage coagulopathy (blood loss due to aortic laceration). (2/08)
- Interpret coagulation studies showing coagulopathy secondary to hypofibrinogenaemia. (1/08)
- Discuss hazards of blood transfusion and blood conservation strategies (radical prostatectomy). (1/08)
- Transfusion strategies for massive blood loss in a child with blunt abdominal trauma. (1/08)
- Massive transfusion management and anaesthesia for damage control surgery (abdominal trauma). (2/07)
- Massive transfusion management in obstetrics. (2/07)
- Discuss the problems of antibodies on cross-matching in a patient who needs urgent transfusion. (2/07)
- What are the treatment options for post-bypass bleeding, including the role of factor VII? (1/07)
- Describe the perioperative management of anticoagulation in emergency spinal cord decompression, including risks of ceasing anticoagulation. (2/06)
- Describe appropriate perioperative blood conservation strategies in revision total hip replacement. (2/06)
- Discuss the perioperative management of anticoagulant therapy in the context of atrial fibrillation and potential blood loss (revision total hip). (2/06)
- Manage major blood loss and discuss the use of the cell saver in obstetrics. (2/06)

Burns

- Resuscitation and initial management of burns/trauma. (2/08)
- Discuss the indications for escharotomy in burns. (2/08)
- Describe the safe management of airway and intubation to a general practitioner with respect to a patient with airway burns and stridor. (2/06)
- Describe the acute management of 50% burns, including analgesia, fluids and retrieval. (2/06)
- Discuss the management of change of dressing for burns patient in the ward. (2/06)

Cardiothoracic anaesthesia

- Diagnose and manage hypoxia during one-lung ventilation. (1/09)
- Describe a safe approach to anaesthesia for laser bronchoscopy. (2/08)
- Preoperative assessment of a patient with a large mediastinal mass. (2/08)
- Discuss strategies for lung separation in a patient with a difficult airway. (1/08)
- Troubleshoot problems with ventilation during one-lung ventilation. (1/08)
- Anaesthetic management of patient with broncho-pleural fistula and empyema following pneumonectomy. (2/07)
- Anaesthesia for thoracoscopic surgery and the management of intraoperative hypotension and problems with ventilation. (2/07)
- Discuss the pathophysiology of aortic stenosis, indications for valve replacement, and optimal timing for surgery (patient has developed pulmonary oedema). (1/07)
- Induction of anaesthesia for severe aortic stenosis with pulmonary oedema. (1/07)
- Management of AF and hypotension in the pre-bypass period. (1/07)
- Discuss an anaesthetic plan and options for surgical repair of injury to thoracic trachea. (1/07)
- Optimise a patient with recent myocardial infarction and cardiogenic shock preoperatively, including placement of intra-aortic balloon pump (IABP). (1/07)
- Describe placement, optimal positioning and timing of IABP. (1/07)
- Describe an approach to patient with anticipated and actual difficulty weaning from bypass (± use of milrinone, levosimendan). (1/07)
- What would your approach be to a request for sedation of a hypotensive, agitated patient with coronary rupture during angioplasty? (1/06)
- A 52-year-old man with failed coronary angioplasty to the left anterior descending artery is transferred to the operating theatre for urgent coronary artery bypass grafting. What are the anaesthetic implications/priorities of this case? (2/05)

Co-existing disease

- Manage acute cardiogenic shock in a patient undergoing urgent coronary stent placement in the cardiac catheter laboratory. (2/09)
- Recognise (ECG) and manage slow AF in the preoperative period. (2/09)
- Understand the Fontan circulation and the principles of haemodynamic management in the perioperative period when the patient presents for appendicectomy. (2/09)
- Manage a patient with an implanted AICD for ECT at a stand-alone psychiatric hospital. (2/09)

- Understand the implications of naltrexone use in the perioperative period (alcohol dependence). (2/09)
- Implications of cancer and its treatment for anaesthesia (metastatic breast cancer). (1/09)
- Manage chronic obstructive pulmonary disease (COPD) perioperatively. (1/09)
- Implications of cancer and its treatment for anaesthesia (child with acute lymphoblastic leukaemia). (1/09)
- Access and manage a potential malignant hyperthermia risk patient. (1/09)
- Manage sepsis in the perioperative period. (1/09)
- Management of severe heart failure, including pharmacological treatment and biventricular pacing. (2/08)
- Resuscitation of haemophiliac with factor VIII inhibitors and chest trauma. (2/08)
- Make an assessment of hepatic disease and optimise condition preoperatively. (2/08)
- Manage perioperative myocardial ischaemia in a patient with coronary stents. (2/08)
- Pharmacology and clinical significance of prolonged QT syndrome, including ECG diagnosis. (2/08)
- Emergency anaesthesia for patient with prolonged QT syndrome (appendicectomy). (2/08)
- Sedation and anaesthesia for patient with severe rheumatoid arthritis. (2/08)
- Undertake appropriate preoperative cardiac risk evaluation in patient with AAA. (1/08)
- Preoperative respiratory assessment of COPD patient. (1/08)
- Principles of treatment of heart failure (in pregnancy). (1/08)
- Describe appropriate perioperative management of a patient with myasthenia gravis for thymectomy. (1/08)
- Implications of rheumatoid arthritis and long-term steroids for anaesthesia/ surgery. (1/08)
- Discuss the preoperative assessment of a diabetic patient. (1/08)
- Preoperative assessment for morbidly obese patient (hip replacement) and plan for anaesthesia including thromboprophylaxis. (2/07)
- Principles of anaesthetic management of a patient with sickle cell disease. (2/07)
- Preoperative assessment of patient with goitre. (2/07)
- Preoperative assessment and management of a patient with coronary stents requiring total knee replacement. (2/07)
- Preoperative assessment of patient with history of amphetamine abuse. (2/07)
- Preoperative assessment of patient with unstable angina requiring semi-urgent surgery. (2/07)
- Discuss the perioperative management of the alcoholic patient. (2/07)
- Alternative methods of induction in a patient with severe needle phobia. (1/07)
- Perioperative management principles when anaesthetising a patient with hypertrophic obstructive cardiomyopathy (HOCM), including assessment of severity. (1/07)
- Outline the signs expected with C5/6, C6/7 disc disease. (1/07)
- Assess cardiovascular risk in a patient due for cataract extraction (stable angina, NIDDM, hypertension, atrial fibrillation (AF)). (1/07)

- Management of anticoagulation in patient with AF for cataract surgery. (1/07)
- Discuss the perioperative care of a patient with opioid addiction. (1/07)
- Preoperative investigation and resuscitation of an elderly patient with peritonitis and Alzheimer's disease. (1/07)
- Assessment of asthma severity and optimise treatment of asthma prior to emergency appendicectomy. (1/07)
- Outline problems with angiotensin-converting enzyme inhibitors and anaesthesia and appropriate interventions for hypotension. (1/07)
- Describe the impact of preoperative chemotherapy on anaesthetic management. (2/06)
- Discuss the perioperative management of phaeochromocytoma. (2/06)
- Describe the preoperative assessment and management of dyspnoea (metastatic carcinoma breast). (2/06)
- Discuss the implications of alternative therapies for anaesthesia. (2/06)
- Manage the issues of alcoholism and anaesthesia. (2/06)
- Fluid resuscitation in an elderly patient with dead gut. (2/06)
- Discuss the perioperative management of carcinoid syndrome. (2/06)
- Discuss the management of a patient with tricuspid incompetence secondary to carcinoid, including cardiovascular monitoring (central venous pressure monitoring vs trans-oesophageal echocardiography). (2/06)
- Safe conduct of anaesthesia for patient with ischaemic heart disease. (2/06)
- Discuss the perioperative management of a patient on steroids. (2/06)
- Preoperative resuscitation of elderly lady with perforated viscus, cardiac failure, COPD, peripheral vascular disease. (2/06)
- Assessment of patient with obstructed inguinal hernia who has a history of chronic renal failure, no dialysis for 4 days and signs of fluid overload. (1/06)
- Shortness of breath in patient with ovarian malignancy and a history of rheumatoid arthritis. (1/06)
- What are the implications of morbid obesity to anaesthesia? (130 kg woman with ischaemic heart disease, lung malignancy for lobectomy) (1/06)
- Preoperative work up for 25-year-old male with severe depression for ECT on tranylcypromine. (1/06)
- Preoperative advice regarding medications (clopidogrel, metoprolol, enalapril, metformin, omeprazole, diclofenac, simvastatin) in a 75-year-old for total knee replacement in 4 weeks. History includes myocardial infarct 5 years ago, NIDDM and well-controlled hypertension. (2/05)
- Clinical assessment of a systolic murmur found at pre-assessment clinic in a 65-year-old for resection of the larynx and free flap. (2/05)
- Perioperative steroid management of 40-year-old woman with Crohn's disease for redo ileostomy, currently on 15 mg/day of prednisolone. She has severe osteoporosis and old fracture of L3. (1/05)
- Plan for blood glucose management in a 45-year-old woman seen by a colleague in the anaesthetic clinic with BMI of 32, NIDDM for 5 years, on metformin, glimepiride, atorvastatin, BSL 16 mmol/L. All medications were omitted on the day of surgery; you meet her for the first time in the anaesthetic bay. (1/05)
- A 66-year-old male presents to the pre-admission clinic 1 week prior to laparoscopic gastric banding. He is on atorvastatin and has sleep apnoea. His observations are: BP 171/101 mmHg, PR 84 b/min, SaO_2 96%, weight 138 kg. What is the significance of his blood pressure? (1/05)

• 54-year-old woman (non-smoker) presenting for vaginal hysterectomy, with 12-year history of multiple sclerosis (Rx beta interferon 8 million units alternate days, paroxetine). Anxious to talk to you about last GA where she vomited for 3 days postoperatively. What do you advise her with respect to her anaesthetic choices and management of her postoperative nausea and vomiting? (1/05)

Complications of anaesthesia
• Diagnose and manage postoperative hepatic dysfunction. (2/09)
• Manage emergence delirium in a developmentally delayed 20-year-old following GA for restorative dental work. (2/09)
• Manage suspected awareness in a child. (1/09)
• Diagnose and manage compartment syndrome in the presence of strong analgesics. (1/09)
• Prevention and management of dental damage following intubation. (2/08)
• Describe diagnosis and management of aspiration. (1/08)
• Different management strategies for post-dural puncture headache and discuss appropriate handling of adverse event. (2/07)
• Manage awareness in patient following caesarean section. (2/07)
• Manage complication (including prevention) of blocking the wrong eye prior to cataract surgery. (1/07)
• Describe the management of a postoperative nerve palsy following total hip replacement. (2/06)

Data interpretation
• Recognise significant tracheal narrowing on imaging (CXR and CT) in patient with retrosternal thyroid. (2/09)
• Interpret and manage electrolyte abnormalities in patient with anorexia nervosa. (1/09)
• Interpret ABG, CXR in obstructive lung disease. (1/09)
• Interpret ECG of patient with heart failure/ischaemic heart disease. (1/09)
• Interpret ECG of cardiac tamponade, atrial fibrillation. (1/09)
• Interpret a preoperative CXR with a pneumothorax. (1/09)
• Interpret and explain electrolyte and acid-base abnormalities in chronic renal failure. (1/09)
• Interpret investigations (especially blood gases) relevant to severe sepsis. (1/09)
• ECG interpretation in ischaemic heart disease. (2/08)
• Interpret CXR showing pulmonary oedema. (1/08)
• ABGs showing mixed respiratory and metabolic acidosis in patient with peritonitis. (1/08)
• Interpretation of respiratory function tests. (1/08)
• Interpret basic echo data. (1/08)
• Interpret and troubleshoot changes in CO_2 traces. (1/08)
• Interpret neuromuscular monitoring and discuss criteria for safe extubation. (1/08)
• Interpret ECG showing WPW. (1/08)
• Interpret ABGs of patient with diabetic ketoacidosis. (1/08)
• ECG with intraoperative AF. (2/07)
• ECG with intraoperative complete heart block. (2/07)
• X-ray of cervical spine with fracture in patient with ankylosing spondylitis. (2/06)
• Interpret ABGs in a patient with dead gut (severe metabolic acidosis). (2/06)

Emergency/crisis situations

- Diagnose (ECG) and manage complete heart block, including the appropriate settings for temporary pacing. (2/09)
- Diagnose and manage an obstructed expiratory valve on the self-inflating bag during transfer to the intensive care unit. (2/09)
- Manage postoperative acute pulmonary oedema. (2/09)
- Manage a total intraoperative power failure. (2/09)
- Recognise (ECG) and manage rapid AF intraoperatively (endoluminal AAA). (2/09)
- Diagnose and manage an obstruction to the expiratory limb of the circle circuit leading to a pneumothorax. (2/09)
- Manage a patient who fails to wake following a prolonged seizure (ECT) at a stand-alone psychiatric hospital. (2/09)
- Manage an intraoperative fire. (2/09)
- Diagnose and manage magnesium toxicity. (2/09)
- Diagnose (including ECG) and manage intraoperative myocardial ischaemia during carotid endarterectomy. (2/09)
- Diagnose and manage acute postoperative cardiac tamponade. (1/09)
- Manage hypertension, tachycardia, ST changes, ventricular tachycardia following adrenaline infiltration. (1/09)
- Diagnose and manage failure to wake postoperatively (cerebral tumour). (1/09)
- Manage postoperative confusion. (1/09)
- Diagnose and manage intraoperative air embolus. (1/09)
- Diagnose and manage VT/VF with a faulty defibrillator. (1/09)
- Manage intraoperative myocardial ischaemia. (1/09)
- Manage difficulties with ventilation intraoperatively (septic patient). (1/09)
- Diagnose and manage hypotension secondary to concealed haemorrhage. (2/08)
- Management of ventilation in face of increasing hypoxia. (2/08)
- Diagnosis and management of hyperkalaemic cardiac arrest. (2/08)
- Management of intraoperative ST changes and ventricular tachycardia. (2/08)
- Management of haemorrhage in radiology and transfer of patient to operating theatre. (2/08)
- Management of failure to wake from general anaesthesia. (2/08)
- Diagnosis and management of anaphylaxis in the prone position. (2/08)
- Management of pulmonary haemorrhage in the coagulopathic patient. (2/08)
- Manage airway obstruction in recovery post-microlaryngoscopy. (2/08)
- Diagnose and treat tension pneumothorax in recovery. (2/08)
- Diagnose and treat pulmonary oedema and coagulopathy (eclampsia). (1/08)
- Discuss the differential diagnosis and management of intraoperative hypoxia. (1/08)
- Describe appropriate differential diagnosis and management of severe hypotension due to reaction to contrast (endoluminal AAA repair). (1/08)
- Describe the differential diagnosis and management of postoperative delirium (alcohol withdrawal). (1/08)
- Differential diagnosis and management of intraoperative hypotension (air embolism in radical prostatectomy). (1/08)
- Intraoperative hypoxia due to pulmonary contusions in a child. (1/08)
- Recognise and manage hypoxia and difficulty with ventilation from misplaced tracheostomy tube. (1/08)

- Discuss differential diagnosis and management of profound hypotension due to cardiac tamponade. (1/08)
- Fluid and electrolyte management of patient with diabetic ketoacidosis. (1/08)
- Differential diagnosis, investigation and management of postoperative cognitive dysfunction (due to stroke). (1/08)
- Intraoperative hypoxia in patient with ARDS and multiple organ failure. (2/07)
- Management of high spinal block, including maternal and fetal resuscitation. (2/07)
- Management of post-thyroidectomy patient with neck haematoma with airway obstruction. (2/07)
- Manage rapid AF intraoperatively. (2/07)
- Recognition and management of complete heart block. (2/07)
- Management of intraoperative hypercarbia during laparoscopy. (2/07)
- Management of postoperative fitting due to hyponatraemia. (2/07)
- Management of intraoperative hypoxia due to pneumothorax or bronchospasm. (2/07)
- Discuss appropriate management of airway fire with airway laser. (2/07)
- Basic and advanced life support for an obese postoperative patient with difficult airway. (2/07)
- Management and investigation following failure to wake postoperatively (carotid endarterectomy). (2/07)
- Diagnose and manage perioperative myocardial infarction. (2/07)
- Management of postoperative airway obstruction in recovery (postoperative cervical fusion). (1/07)
- Management plan for failed intubation in an infant. (1/07)
- Systematic approach to a fall in $ETCO_2$ in a patient in the sitting position. (1/07)
- Differential diagnosis and management of intraoperative hypoxia (dental case in child). (1/07)
- Differential diagnosis and management of hypotension and difficulty with ventilation in asthmatic undergoing laparoscopy (anaphylaxis). (1/07)
- List the differential diagnosis and describe the management of intraoperative hypotension. (2/06)
- Discuss the differential diagnosis of tension pneumothorax intraoperatively. (2/06)
- Describe the differential diagnosis and management of fat/tumour embolism. (2/06)
- Describe the management of rapid AF intraoperatively. (2/06)
- Detect and manage local anaesthetic toxicity. (2/06)
- Causes of inadequate reversal, including the role of neuromuscular monitoring. (2/06)

ENT/maxillofacial/thyroid surgery
- Anaesthetic technique for microlaryngoscopy in patient with ischaemic heart disease, diabetes and supraglottic tumour. (2/08)
- Induction of anaesthesia for bleeding post-tonsillectomy. (2/08)
- Assessment and anaesthetic plan for 17-year-old autistic boy with dental abscess. (1/08)
- Differential diagnosis of stridor (painful, 2-day onset) in 35-year-old. (1/08)

- Preoperative assessment of patient for laser surgery to the larynx. Discuss with appropriate decision-making the issues relevant to laser surgery involving the larynx and trachea. (2/07)
- Provide advice to a colleague on how to anaesthetise a 45-year-old, 112 kg patient for septoplasty and FESS. He is a smoker with obstructive sleep apnoea. (1/06)
- A 43-year-old depressed (on moclobemide) smoker with a history of awareness and PONV presents for revision mastoidectomy with facial nerve monitoring. List the main issues of the anaesthesia. (2/05)
- Preoperative assessment of 45-year-old woman with large multinodular goitre with retrosternal extension presenting for subtotal thyroidectomy. (2/05)
- Preoperative assessment of a 45-year-old, 112 kg patient for septoplasty and FESS. He is a smoker with obstructive sleep apnoea. (1/05)

Equipment/environment
- Describe and justify your anaesthetic machine check. (1/08)
- Describe the minimum standards required for anaesthesia in the electro-physiology lab. (1/08)

General surgery
- Discuss the options for sedation/anaesthesia for patient for PEG insertion (motor neurone disease). (1/08)
- Optimisation of the patient for oesophagectomy. (2/07)
- Induction and post-induction resuscitation in patient with peritonitis and large bowel obstruction. (1/07)
- Anaesthetic plan for oesophageal surgery in patient with previous awareness due to drug error. (1/07)
- Discuss open vs laparoscopic approach to appendicectomy in patient with severe asthma and peritonitis. (1/07)
- Describe and manage the problems of laparoscopic surgery (adrenalectomy for phaeochromocytoma). (2/06)
- Discuss the perioperative management of a patient for major liver resection with carcinoid. (2/06)
- Discuss a safe choice of anaesthesia for elderly patient with a perforated viscus. (2/06)
- Anaesthetic issues for 75-year-old man with carcinoma of the oesophagus for oesophagectomy via right thoracotomy. (2/05)

Intensive care
- Manage difficulties with ventilation in a patient with severe chest trauma. (2/09)
- Discuss the diagnosis of brain death. (2/08)
- Management of the patient for organ donation. (2/08)
- Intubation of 11-year-old child for deteriorating severe asthma in a rural hospital. (1/06)

Neurosurgical anaesthesia
- Conduct safe neuroanaesthesia in the presence of significant co-morbidities (secondary cerebral metastasis, previous pneumonectomy). (2/09)
- Diagnose and manage acute spinal cord injury, including spinal shock. (1/09)

- Manage a seizure following head injury. (1/09)
- Induction of anaesthesia in morbidly obese, unco-operative patient with frontal lobe tumour. (1/09)
- Manage intracranial pressure pre- and intra-operatively. (1/09)
- Manage sub-arachnoid haemorrhage (SAH) perioperatively in the context of coiling in the radiology suite. (1/09)
- Diagnose and manage a ruptured aneurysm during coiling. (1/09)
- Resuscitation and management of patient with raised intracranial pressure. (2/08)
- Principles of maintaining spinal cord perfusion in patient with spinal cord compression. (2/08)
- Describe appropriate initial assessment and resuscitation in 2-year-old child with head injury. (1/08)
- Discuss strategies to control raised intracranial pressure. (1/08)
- Describe a safe technique for anaesthesia for decompressive craniectomy in 2-year-old child. (1/08)
- Management of trauma patient with rapidly deteriorating GCS and principles of cerebral protection. (2/07)
- Anaesthesia for CT and halo traction for 15-year-old intellectually impaired child with C1-2 fracture-dislocation. (2/07)
- Discuss the principles of spinal cord protection and monitoring. (2/07)
- Discuss anaesthesia for urgent spinal cord decompression (quadriplegic post halo). (2/07)
- Recognise significance of patient's neurological signs prior to cervical decompression in patient with canal stenosis. (1/07)
- Pros and cons of prone vs sitting position for posterior cervical decompressive laminectomy. (1/07)
- Safe plan for anaesthesia in the sitting position. (1/07)
- Discuss the diagnosis and management of a spontaneous epidural haematoma. (2/06)
- Issues of anaesthesia for emergency spinal cord decompression, including maintenance of spinal cord perfusion. (2/06)
- Plan anaesthesia for cervical spine stabilisation and fusion, including intubation issues (ankylosing spondylitis with fracture). (2/06)
- Issues of prone positioning in a patient with an unstable cervical spine. (2/06)
- Discuss the role of spinal cord monitoring. (2/06)
- Plan for safe extubation following cervical fusion in ankylosing spondylitis. (2/06)
- Demonstrate an understanding of the effects of rebleeding in subarachnoid haemorrhage. (2/06)
- How do you grade patients who present with aneurysmal subarachnoid haemorrhage? (2/05)

Obstetrics and gynaecology
- Assess the febrile pregnant woman with prolonged ruptured membranes. (2/09)
- Discuss epidural analgesia in the presence of maternal fever. (2/09)
- Manage sepsis during caesarean section. (2/09)
- Diagnose and manage a seizure during labour. (2/09)

- Manage a cardiac arrest during pregnancy (secondary to magnesium overdose). (2/09)
- Apply EMST principles to pregnant patient and assess abdominal pain following trauma. (1/09)
- Manage intra-abdominal haemorrhage at caesarean section. (1/09)
- Manage an obstetric and neonatal emergency in a hospital without obstetric service. (1/09)
- Manage severe bleeding at caesarean section requiring hysterectomy. (1/09)
- Management of cocaine toxic patient for caesarean section with placental abruption. (2/08)
- Manage failed intubation in obese patient requiring general anaesthesia for caesarean section. (2/08)
- Plan for general anaesthesia in malignant hyperthermia-susceptible woman requiring caesarean section. (2/08)
- Prenatal advice to woman at risk of malignant hyperthermia regarding analgesic options for labour and delivery. (2/08)
- Describe appropriate assessment and resuscitation of a woman presenting with eclampsia. (1/08)
- Discuss options for anaesthesia for woman presenting for emergency caesarean section (eclampsia). (1/08)
- Differential diagnosis of initial presentation of dyspnoea in pregnancy (heart failure). (1/08)
- Anaesthetic plan (regional vs general) for caesarean section, including monitoring and postoperative recovery, for woman with heart failure. (1/08)
- Describe an approach to obtaining consent for epidural analgesia in labour. (2/07)
- Anaesthetic management for caesarean section of 32-week gestation woman with placenta praevia and large ante-partum haemorrhage. (2/07)
- Management of intraoperative haemorrhage due to placenta praevia. (2/07)
- Anaesthetic assessment of morbidly obese parturient, including deciding optimum place and timing of delivery. (1/07)
- Management of emergency caesarean section in morbidly obese parturient. (1/07)
- Assessment, differential diagnosis and management of severe unstable hypertension in pregnancy. (1/07)
- Safely manage general anaesthesia in the setting of severe unstable hypertension in pregnancy; manage unstable haemodynamics intraoperatively. (1/07)
- Management alternatives for above if patient had been known to have phaeochromocytoma before caesarean section. (1/07)
- Discuss the induction and management of general anaesthesia in pregnancy (appendicitis at 32 weeks). (2/06)
- Discuss the maintenance of uteroplacental flow and fetal monitoring. (2/06)
- Manage fetal bradycardia intraoperatively. (2/06)
- Conduct the initial assessment and resuscitation of the pregnant trauma patient. (2/06)
- Discuss management of hypotension, uteroplacental blood flow and fetal protection in an out-of-theatre environment (abdominal trauma). (2/06)
- Describe a safe anaesthetic plan for laparotomy/caesarean section for above. (2/06)

- Immediate management of a 32-year-old being induced at 41 weeks who collapses shortly after her membranes are ruptured. (1/06)
- Differential diagnosis of shortness of breath in 26-year-old primiparous woman presenting at 38 weeks. (1/06)
- 32-year-old obese multigravida (seventh pregnancy) for repeat elective caesarean section with low-lying placenta. What obstetric history would you obtain? (2/05)
- A 34-year-old primigravida with functioning epidural at 5–6 cm in OP position. Obstetrician wishes to perform urgent caesarean section, but all theatres are occupied with elective cases. How do you respond to the obstetrician's request? (2/05)
- Anaesthetic issues in an otherwise well 42-year-old with history of PONV, ceased OCP 3 months ago for lap-assisted vaginal hysterectomy; expected to be a long case. (1/05)
- Further management of healthy nulliparous woman with BMI 40 requiring caesarean section for class 2 fetal compromise. Following a difficult spinal insertion, block has spread to T9 after 25 minutes. (1/05)
- A 39-year-old at 15 weeks pregnant booked with a diagnosis of ruptured ectopic pregnancy. Medications include folate, salbutamol and some natural health supplements. What specific questions would you ask the gynaecologist when she books the case? (1/05)

Orthopaedics

- Discuss regional anaesthesia, including anatomy, for open reduction, internal fixation of fractured humeral head. (1/09)
- Manage severe hypoxia and hypotension during femoral/acetabular cement application. (1/09)
- Discuss the risks and benefits of regional anaesthesia for fractured neck of femur. (2/08)
- Management of intraoperative hypotension following reaming and cementing in total hip. (2/07)
- Problems associated with knee replacement surgery and alternative anaesthetic techniques. (2/07)
- DVT prophylaxis for patient undergoing ankle reconstruction (obese smoker). (1/07)
- Outline positioning problems for 100 kg patient undergoing arthroscopic acromioplasty. (1/07)
- What are the issues relating to revision hip replacement for a patient with longstanding AF and transient ischaemic attacks prior to being put on warfarin? (2/06)
- Discuss the safe use of a tourniquet. (2/06)
- A 12-year-old girl for correction of scoliosis and instrumented posterior spinal fusion, with prone position surgery, expected to take 4–6 hours. What findings from your preoperative assessment would make you consider elective postoperative ventilation for this patient? (2/05)
- What positions are used for shoulder arthroscopy? What problems could you anticipate from these positions? (25-year-old elite athlete for day surgery in beach chair position) (2/05)
- Anaesthetic options for closed reduction of Colles' fracture in frail 75-year-old alcoholic with COPD, hypertension and depression. (1/05)

Paediatric anaesthesia

- Assess a medically unwell child with pneumonia who requires drainage of a large pleural effusion. (2/09)
- Manage severe oxygen desaturation in the ward (including ABG interpretation in the child above). (2/09)
- Manage intra-hospital transfer of the child above to radiology for pleural drainage. (2/09)
- Manage basic resuscitation in a 2-year-old child following near drowning. (2/09)
- Diagnose and manage resistant VF in a near drowning. (2/09)
- Diagnose and manage persistent hypoxia in near drowning (including interpretation of ABG). (2/09)
- Induction of anaesthesia in unfasted child with difficult IV access. (1/09)
- Manage neonatal resuscitation. (1/09)
- Options for IV access and fluid resuscitation in bleeding post-tonsillectomy. (2/08)
- Management of neonatal resuscitation. (2/08)
- Resuscitation of infant with dehydration secondary to obstructed inguinal hernia. (2/08)
- Induction of anaesthesia for infant with bowel obstruction. (2/08)
- Discuss options for IV access in a child (difficult veins). (1/08)
- Principles of conservative vs operative management of blunt abdominal trauma in children. (1/08)
- Discuss anaesthesia and postoperative analgesia for laparoscopy in children and problems posed by obesity. (2/07)
- Postoperative fluid management in children. (2/07)
- Management in the emergency department of 20-month-old child with hypoxia and inhaled foreign body. (2/07)
- Anaesthetic management of child with inhaled foreign body. (2/07)
- Discuss criteria for day surgery in infants (2.9 kg, inguinal hernia). (1/07)
- Pros and cons for spinal vs GA for infant having inguinal hernia repair. (1/07)
- Preoperative assessment of child with upper respiratory infection with practical decision criteria for cancellation or not. (1/07)
- Appropriate technique for dental anaesthesia in children, including nasal intubation. (1/07)
- Discharge criteria for day surgery in children (dental case). (1/07)
- Deal with an anxious child and family for major surgery. (2/06)
- Discuss major blood loss and perioperative fluid management in children, including allowable blood loss, transfusion thresholds. (2/06)
- Describe neonatal resuscitation. (2/06)
- Describe a sensitive approach to parental presence or absence at induction. (2/06)
- Describe the use of desflurane and a circle system in children. (2/06)
- Anxious child with cerebral palsy requiring dental extractions under general anaesthesia. (1/06)
- Anaesthetic concerns with a 4-year-old boy with progressive weakness and muscle wasting for muscle biopsy. (2/05)
- Request to resuscitate a neonate while administering GA for caesarean section to the mother. Calculate Apgar score. Baby has irregular respirations, centrally cyanosed, grimaces during suction, limp and not moving, PR 90. (1/05)

- A 4-year-old child with Down syndrome presents to day surgery unit for tonsillectomy and adenoidectomy. The parents say the child is often 'chesty', has frequent respiratory tract infections, snores and is needle phobic. On auscultation you detect a murmur. How will you assess the significance of this murmur? (1/05)
- An 8-year-old child with cystic fibrosis with worsening chest infection presents for insertion of a portacath (21 kg, difficult IV access, has none at present; saturation is 91%, sputum growing *Burkholderia cepacia*). What is cystic fibrosis and what are the significant anaesthetic issues in this patient who requires a general anaesthetic for insertion of a portacath? (1/05)

Pain management

- Formulate a perioperative pain management plan in a patient for acromioplasty, who is taking oxycodone and refuses regional analgesia. (2/09)
- Manage severe pain in the recovery ward (patient above). (2/09)
- Manage severe pain from compound fracture of tibia/fibula not responsive to initial treatment. (2/09)
- Manage postoperative pain following pleurodesis. (1/09)
- Manage postoperative pain (child with fractures developing compartment syndrome) with increasing analgesic requirements. (1/09)
- Pain management in opioid tolerant patient undergoing major surgery (multilevel posterior fusion). (2/08)
- Analgesia for mastectomy and chronic post-surgical pain. (2/08)
- Management of postoperative neuropathic pain following spinal cord decompression. (2/08)
- Describe pain management options in thoracotomy, including use of paravertebral catheters. (1/08)
- Postoperative pain management in patient with back surgery/opioid use following radical prostatectomy. (1/08)
- Discuss pain management options following sternotomy. (1/08)
- Discuss appropriate perioperative pain management in patient on long-term opioids. (1/08)
- Alternatives for pain management following total hip replacement. (2/07)
- Pain management in opioid tolerant patient with poor response to prescribed analgesia. (2/07)
- Pain management options in patient with thoracotomy for bronchopleural fistula and empyema. (2/07)
- Approach to pain management in an obese post-bowel resection patient with sleep apnoea. (2/07)
- Evaluate postoperative pain management options for oesophagectomy. (2/07)
- Discuss pain management in a patient on chronic opioids (prostate cancer, COPD, vertebral metastases, rib fractures following fall). (1/07)
- Treatment options for neuropathic pain including systemic treatments and the risks and benefits of intrathecal therapy. (1/07)
- Anaesthesia and postoperative pain management of a patient with opioid addiction. (1/07)
- Discuss issues around patient-controlled analgesia (PCA) usage in patients absenting themselves from a ward. (1/07)
- Postoperative analgesia for acromioplasty including interscalene block. (1/07)
- Discuss the anaesthetic management of a patient on naltrexone. (2/06)

- Discuss the advantages and disadvantages of an epidural for postoperative analgesia (laparotomy and bowel resection for Crohn's disease). (2/06)
- Uncontrolled pain in a nurse who had ORIF of fractured radius and ulna the previous day. (1/06)
- Management of postoperative pain in diabetic post below-knee amputation, burning and unresponsive to morphine. (1/06)
- Diabetic 65-year-old with moderate renal impairment (Cr 0.18 mmol/L) with fractured ribs and ankle has difficulty breathing and chest wall pain. What are the initial issues you would deal with when you see her? (2/05)
- A 37-year-old man with a compound tibial fracture and a past history of IV drug abuse, current medications methadone 80 mg/day, diazepam 5 mg TDS prn, oxycodone 20 mg BD prn. A lumbar epidural (for post-op analgesia) was easily placed prior to GA and the procedure has been completed uneventfully. What are your instructions to the recovery nurses regarding observations required for this epidural? (1/05)

Regional anaesthesia

- Understand the risks and benefits of neuraxial blockade for postoperative analgesia in patients receiving intraoperative anticoagulation (endoluminal AAA). (2/09)
- Describe a regional technique (including relevant anatomy) for pain management in a patient with a compound fractured tibia/fibula. (2/09)
- Describe a regional technique (including relevant anatomy) for carotid endarterectomy. (2/09)
- Discuss regional anaesthesia for arterio-venous fistula formation in chronic renal failure patient, including relevant anatomy. (1/09)
- Regional anaesthesia options for inguinal hernia repair and innervation of the inguinal region. (1/08)
- Options for regional anaesthesia for ankle arthrodesis in patient with rheumatoid arthritis and back pain, and describe the innervation of the ankle. (1/08)
- Technique for regional blockade for carotid endarterectomy. (2/07)
- Postoperative analgesia for ankle reconstruction, including appropriate local anaesthesia technique. (1/07)
- Relative merits of sub-tenons vs peribulbar block for cataract surgery, including management of complications. (1/07)
- Discuss consent issues for interscalene block. (1/07)
- Diagnose and manage compartment syndrome in a patient with regional anaesthesia. (2/06)
- Describe the safe use/risks/benefits of continuous brachial plexus block. (2/06)
- Describe the safe use of caudal block (2-year-old for ureteric implant). (2/06)
- Manage epidural problems/failure postoperatively. (2/06)
- Anaesthesia choice for an 83-year-old male with emphysema and a right compound supracondylar fracture of the elbow. You are considering regional blockade (FEV$_1$ 0.75L, CCF, PO$_2$ 58, PCO$_2$ 46). What technique would you choose and why? (1/05)

Remote locations

- Manage the transfer of a heavily sedated postoperative patient to another hospital (from day surgery unit). (2/09)

- Manage resuscitation in the MRI suite. (2/08)
- Discuss options for anaesthesia/sedation for electrophysiology studies. (1/08)
- Priorities for providing sedation for colonoscopy in 65-year-old man with rectal bleeding in a free-standing day surgery unit. (1/06)
- Priorities following an urgent request to provide sedation for anxious patient in the MRI scanner having a cranial scan (patient already in scanner). (2/05)
- Response to call from intern regarding unconscious 25-year-old with stridor in ward following admission for observation following head injury. You are in the middle of an open appendicectomy. (2/05)
- Request to anaesthetise 120 kg woman in catheter lab for pacemaker/implantable defibrillator, with myocardial infarct 8 months ago. What would you ask the cardiologist?(1/05)
- You are new to a hospital and are phoned by a gastroenterologist wanting you to anaesthetise a 70-year-old diabetic for an urgent ERCP. What specific information do you discuss with the endoscopist about the case? (1/05)

Trauma

- Manage multiple trauma with severe bleeding in accident victim with major abdominal and pelvic injuries. (2/09)
- Resuscitate a 20-year-old patient with blunt chest trauma (EMST principles) and manage a large haemopneumothorax. (2/09)
- Manage severe trauma (EMST guidelines to head/neck injury and near drowning). (1/09)
- Initial assessment and resuscitation of child with abdominal trauma. (1/08)
- Discuss the early (emergency department) management of exsanguinating blunt abdominal trauma. (2/07)
- Discuss the management of the cervical spine in a patient with severe head injury. Discuss clearance of the cervical spine. (2/07)
- ICP monitoring during surgery; management of ICP changes. (2/07)
- Timing of femoral fixation in trauma patient with raised ICP. (2/07)
- Management of crush injury (28-year-old crushed by forklift), including management of cardiac arrest during reperfusion. (2/07)
- Discuss the problems and describe safe anaesthetic management during transport, embolisation in the angiography suite and application of external fixateurs. (2/07)
- Discuss initial assessment and resuscitation of patient with penetrating chest/mediastinal injury (gunshot wound). Using knowledge of anatomy, outline potentially injured structures. (1/07)
- Describe a safe plan for anaesthesia/analgesia for a patient entrapped by the arm, requiring amputation on site. (2/06)
- Discuss issues involved in anaesthesia for reimplantation of the forearm. (2/06)
- Discuss the issues of out-of-theatre/off-the-floor neurovascular procedures (aneurysm coiling with history of ischaemic heart disease). (2/06)
- Preparation for the arrival of trauma (motorcycle rider, high-speed collision, damage to front of helmet, uncooperative and combative, tachycardia). (1/06)
- Management of 16-year-old girl following fall and trampling by a horse (GCS 15, now 11, facial bruising, tender abdomen). (1/06)
- Priorities in assessment of a patient involved in high speed MVA. At scene, conscious and complaining of pain down left side of body. On arrival, restless but conscious, HR 125, BP 100/60, RR 30, SaO_2 92% on 6 L/min. (1/06)

- Asked to see 26-year-old following high speed MVA with GCS of 10 with chest drain in situ for left haemothorax. Describe the Glasgow coma scale. (2/05)
- Immediate management priorities in a 55-year-old involved in tractor accident with multiple injuries. (1/05)
- Emergency management of a 26-year-old man with multiple stab wounds, including three to the left chest, BP 85/60, RR 40/min, PR 130/min, decreased air entry on the left, unable to record saturation. (1/05)

Vascular surgery

- Compare the risks and benefits of regional versus general anaesthesia for carotid endarterectomy. (2/09)
- Pros and cons of regional vs general anaesthesia for peripheral vascular surgery. (1/09)
- Anaesthetic technique for endoluminal repair of AAA in angiography suite. (1/08)
- Advantages and disadvantages of regional vs general anaesthesia for carotid endarterectomy. (2/07)
- Describe appropriate management of seizure during carotid cross-clamping. (2/07)
- Anaesthesia for femoro-popliteal bypass in patient with unstable angina. (2/07)
- Discuss principles of maintaining graft perfusion perioperatively. (2/06)
- Preoperative management of 65-year-old diabetic with chronic renal failure managed with peritoneal dialysis with ST segment depression in septal leads presenting for femoro-popliteal bypass. (2/05)

Welfare and professional issues

- Discuss the ethical issues surrounding a decision to operate in the face of a poor prognosis (craniotomy to remove an isolated metastasis from lung carcinoma). (2/09)
- Discuss an iatrogenic complication with the patient and family. (2/09)
- Assess a new hospital with a view to providing anaesthesia services for ECT. (2/09)
- Manage difficulties in obtaining consent in 16-year-old with psychiatric problems. (1/09)
- Negotiate a perioperative plan with a Jehovah's Witness patient (placenta praevia). (1/09)
- Manage unprofessional and dangerous behaviour in a colleague. (1/09)
- Management of a needle stick injury to trainee from known hepatitis B carrier. (2/08)
- Discuss the implications of 'Not for Resuscitation' orders for anaesthesia and surgery. (2/08)
- Diagnose/manage/follow-up an iatrogenic drug swap. (2/08)
- Response and understanding of the issues involved in patient request not to be resuscitated in case of life-threatening complications (patient with motor neurone disease). (1/08)
- Discuss issues of further surgery or palliation in end-of-life situation. (1/08)
- Describe the objectives of in-training assessment. (1/08)
- Describe an appropriate plan for assessment of a third-year anaesthesia trainee. (1/08)

- Recognise the signs of possible drug abuse in a colleague and describe appropriate short-term strategy for dealing with the issue. (1/08)
- Management of suspected opioid abuse in a colleague. (2/07)
- Consent in a 39-year-old woman with intellectual impairment. (2/07)
- Appropriate approach for dealing with an impaired colleague. (2/07)
- Strategies for dealing with opioid addicted patient, including community (drug and alcohol, methadone provider). (1/07)
- Implications for anaesthesia of Alzheimer's disease patient, including consent issues. (1/07)
- Describe an appropriate professional and ethical approach to management of syringe swap error (relaxant instead of midazolam). (1/07)
- Discuss reasons for drug errors, including system errors. (1/07)
- Discuss ethical issues around whether to operate on elderly patient with dead gut. (2/06)
- Discuss institutional policy on minimising epidural risk/consequences of epidural haematoma and infection. (2/06)
- Formulate a plan for situation of no available ICU bed and emergency laparotomy in elderly patient with multiple co-morbidities. (2/06)
- Advice to inexperienced registrar for intoxicated patient requiring prolonged orthopaedic procedure. (2/06)

Chapter 6

Data interpretation for the final examination

Never trust anything that can think for itself if you can't see where it keeps its brain.

J K ROWLING

Overview

Prior to 2007 one of three clinical medical vivas in the final FANZCA examination was solely devoted to the interpretation of clinical data. This viva required rapid spot diagnosis of radiographs, electrocardiographs, spirometry results, arterial blood gases and biochemical data (among others), and usually involved a flurry of X-rays and papers to and fro across the examination table. One of the major changes in format of the clinical examination in 2007 was the restructuring of the clinical viva process and removal of this medical viva as an isolated entity. However, candidates should not regard interpretation of investigations as any less critical to their exam preparation. Any commonly used data modality may appear in any section of the examination. Multiple choice questions using biochemical data and ECG features are very common; recent years have seen the appearance of several short-answer written questions that specifically relate to interpretation of test results. Most commonly, candidates are asked to interpret such data in the clinical vivas, either as a component of a clinical scenario given in an anaesthesia viva, or as part of the assessment of a patient in the medical vivas. The advantage of using these latter clinical formats is that they give candidates the opportunity to correlate facets of a clinical situation, or features elicited on history and examination, with appropriate medical investigations.

Always consider the clinical scenario before you, and keep the following questions in mind when reviewing clinical tests: Is this the most appropriate investigation in this situation? How will the results of the test influence my management? Does my interpretation of the test result correlate with the clinical picture? Does the test result solve a clinical problem or raise new concerns?

It is expected that candidates will possess reasonable proficiency at reviewing common modalities and frequently encountered conditions. When faced with a baffling radiograph or ECG it is not appropriate in the examination to defer to the opinion of a radiologist or electrophysiologist. In such situations a comprehensive system for examining each of these is vital and may provide insight that was lacking on initial perusal of the test. The need to practise a technique for reviewing and verbalising results of data interpretation cannot be overemphasised. Many hospitals have libraries of X-rays and ECGs, which in conjunction with major relevant texts provide an invaluable resource.

This chapter contains a discussion of commonly encountered investigations and several clinical examples, including practice cases with the types of questions that might be expected in the exam (for which answers or descriptions are given in the last section of this chapter, commencing on page 192). A comprehensive description of all pathologies that may be encountered is obviously beyond the scope of this book and candidates are urged to read widely around all of these topics in relevant dedicated texts. It is also useful to obtain tutorials from other specialists, such as radiologists and cardiologists, to improve your approach to investigations.

1. Electrocardiography

Interpreting electrocardiographs (ECGs) is a critical skill required of the anaesthetist. It is presumed that candidates understand the physiological principles of ECG generation, and expected that they are familiar with a wide range of ECG abnormalities that may be encountered perioperatively. Be mindful that an ECG in the examination (and in real life) may contain more than one abnormality.

A system for assessing the ECG is useful when no obvious abnormality exists on initial perusal of the trace, or when the trace is unusually complicated with multiple pathological processes. One such system is presented in Box 6.1 (overleaf).

It is possible to describe the ECG to the examiners using the format of a comprehensive system (which can also be a stalling tactic while desperately searching for a hidden abnormality). However, you may be interrupted and asked to comment on an obvious abnormal feature. You should also be aware that commonly generated computer indices (such as axis, QRS duration and segment lengths) are very likely to appear on the ECG tracings you receive in the examination (as they usually do in real life). A computer-generated diagnosis will most probably be deleted.

Always consider the ECG in conjunction with the clinical situation presented or the patient you have seen, all of which may provide clues to help your interpretation of the trace. Similarly, use the information you gain from the ECG to comment on likely diagnoses and required treatment options for that patient.

Some examples of clinical scenarios and associated ECG traces are provided in the following pages. Brief answers to these appear on pages 192–94.

BOX 6.1 Systematic assessment of the ECG

1. Demographic and technical aspects
   - Patient details, date and time
   - Tracing speed (normally 25 mm/s)
   - Tracing amplitude (normally 10 mm/mV)

2. Computer-generated data
   - Axis
   - Segment intervals
   - Heart rate
   - Diagnoses (may be misleading)

3. Rate and rhythm
   - Approximate heart rate is 300 divided by the number of large (0.2 sec) squares between successive R waves
   - Rhythm may be regular, regularly irregular or irregularly irregular
   - Take particular note of the relationship of P waves and QRS complexes (are both always present and related?)

4. Cardiac axis
   - Computer-generated value may be given
   - Downward overall deflection in lead I implies right axis deviation
   - Downward overall deflection in all inferior leads implies left axis deviation
   - Axis determination is frequently useful, even diagnostic

5. Interval duration
   - PR interval normally 0.12–0.2 sec
   - QRS complex duration normally <0.12 sec
   - Corrected QT interval normally <0.44 sec (QTc = QT/$\sqrt{\text{R–R}}$)

6. Individual wave morphology
   - P waves (inverted, bifid, peaked, biphasic)
   - QRS complexes (height, morphology and duration; ectopy; R wave progression)
   - T waves (inversion, amplitude, pseudonormalisation)

7. Segments
   - Assess duration, take-off points and segment heights if divergent from baseline
   - PR segment depression (pericarditis) or elevation (atrial infarct)
   - ST segment depression or elevation

8. Accessory waves and unusual features
   - U waves (hypokalaemia)
   - J waves (hypothermia)
   - Delta waves (accessory pathways)
   - Pacing spikes (single or dual, timing)
   - Saw-tooth baseline (atrial flutter or Parkinsonian tremor)

Case 1

A 15-year-old child presents with intermittent dizziness and palpitations, present when the following ECG was taken:

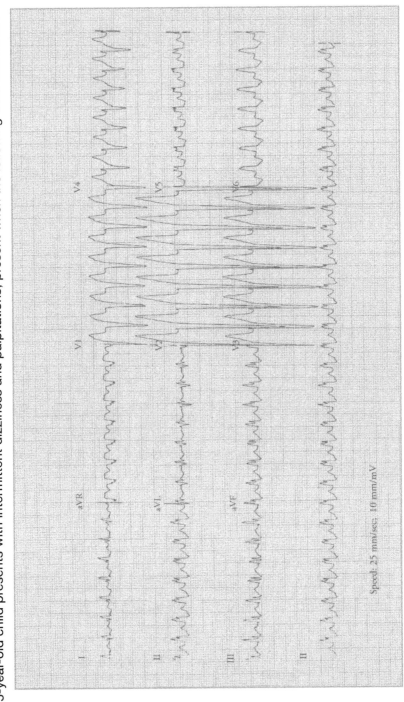

FIGURE 6.1

a Please interpret the ECG.
b What is your differential diagnosis?
c Outline your immediate management of this patient.

Case 1 (cont'd)

Two hours later, the following ECG was obtained from the same patient:

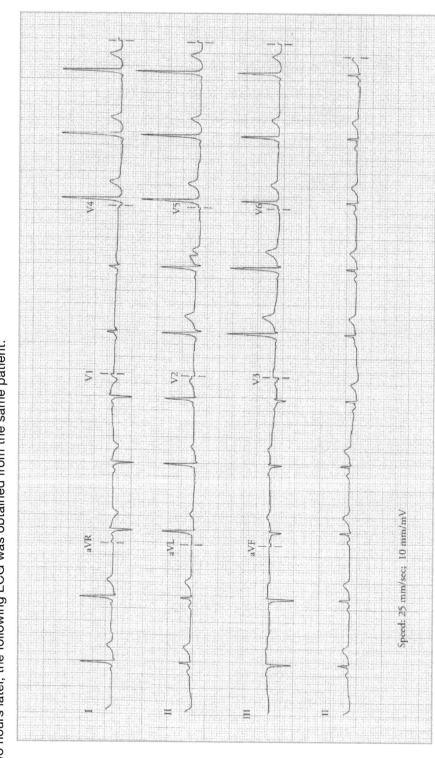

FIGURE 6.2

d What is your diagnosis?

Case 2

A 65-year-old woman presents with exertional chest pain, dizziness and dyspnoea. Her pulse rate is regular, 75 beats/min. She has a loud ejection systolic murmur which radiates to her neck. You ask to see a 12-lead ECG, which appears as follows:

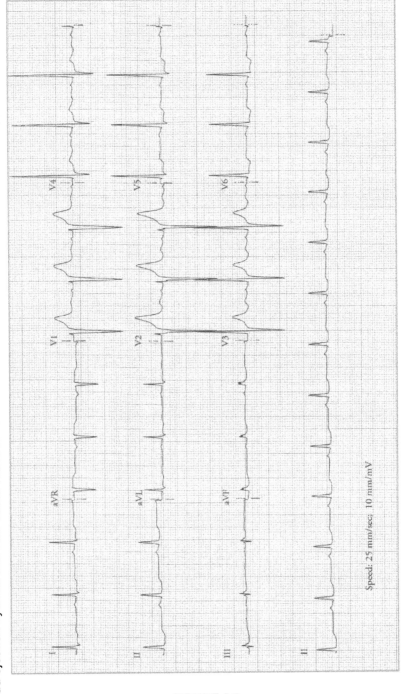

FIGURE 6.3

a Comment on the ECG. Is it consistent with your provisional diagnosis?
b What other investigations would you like to see?

Case 3

A 75-year-old man is seen in preparation for a trans-urethral resection of his prostate. He mentions that he has become increasingly unsteady on his feet. The following routine ECG has been taken:

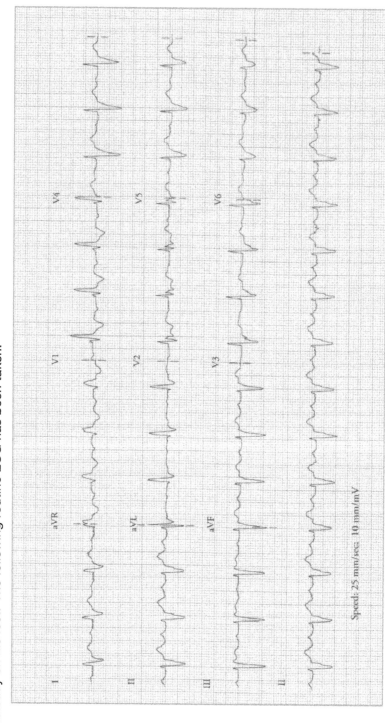

FIGURE 6.4

a Comment on abnormal features of the ECG. Can you make an electrophysiological diagnosis?
b Do you have any concerns about the proposed surgery? Outline your management of this patient.

Case 4

You are called to see a 60-year-old, 115 kg patient who is experiencing chest pain in recovery following an otherwise uneventful laparoscopic cholecystectomy. The patient has a history of pacemaker insertion 5 years previously and smokes 75 cigarettes per day. You arrive as the following ECG is being printed out:

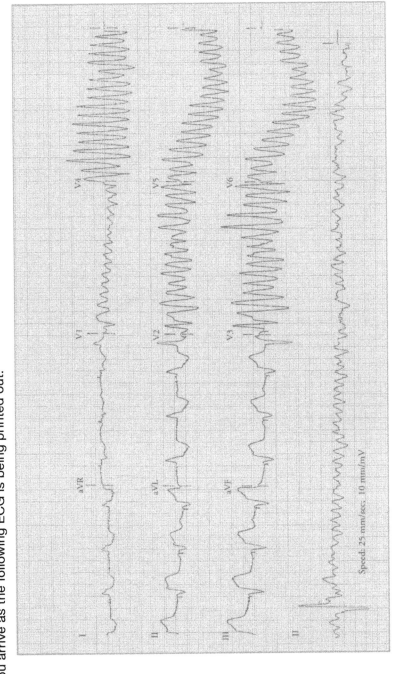

FIGURE 6.5

a Comment on the ECG. What do you think has happened?
b How do you manage this situation?

Case 5

Two days after right hemicolectomy for adenocarcinoma, a 48-year-old patient complains of sudden onset of dyspnoea and chest pain. The following ECG was taken:

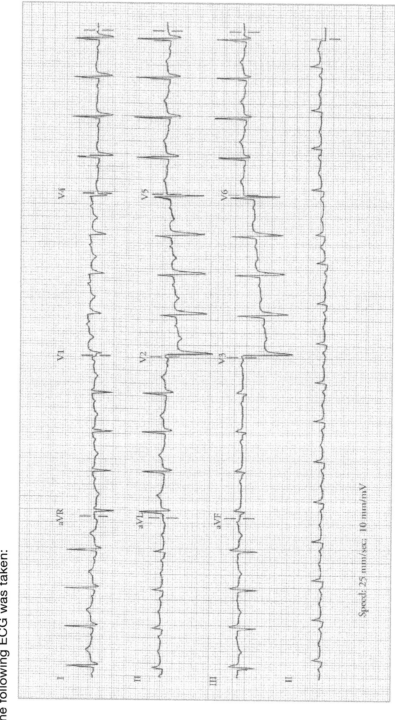

FIGURE 6.6

a What is your differential diagnosis?
b Does the ECG above provide any clues to the diagnosis?
c What further investigations do you require in this patient?

Case 6

A healthy 26-year-old male athlete collapses 7 km into the run leg of the state triathlon championship. On arrival in hospital he is unconscious. An ECG tracing taken in the emergency department appears as follows:

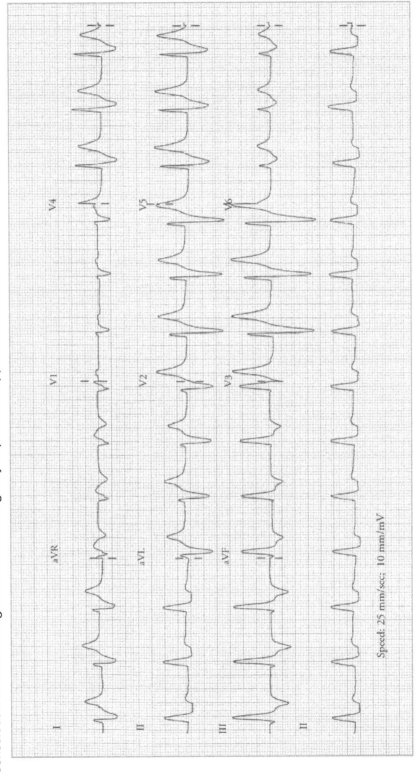

FIGURE 6.7

a Describe the ECG abnormalities present. What is the likely diagnosis?

Case 6 (cont'd)

Twenty minutes later the following ECG trace is obtained:

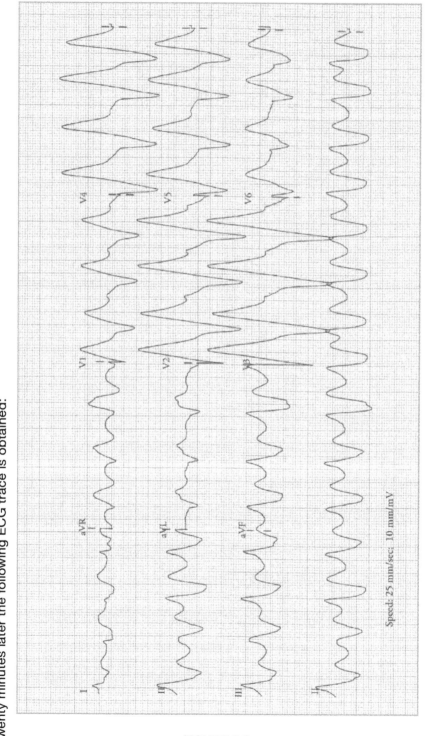

FIGURE 6.8

b Describe the ECG. What do you think has happened?

c Outline your treatment priorities for this patient, including other investigations you might require.

Case 7

A fit, healthy, 18-year-old male presents to pre-admission clinic 2 weeks before undergoing endoscopic sinus surgery. He has a vague recollection of a heart problem in childhood, but is unsure of the details. A 12-lead ECG is obtained:

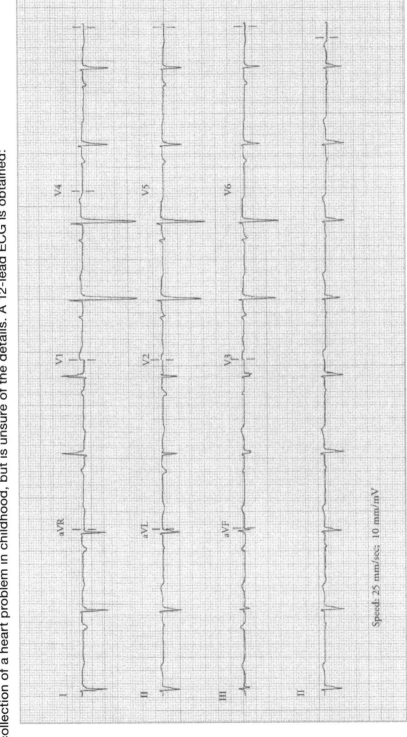

FIGURE 6.9

a Comment on any abnormalities present in this trace. What is the diagnosis?
b Are there any further investigations you would like to see?

Case 8

A 6-year-old child presents for adenotonsillectomy. On examination he looks well, but you hear an ejection systolic murmur at the apex. The nurse on the ward has helpfully provided you with the following ECG trace:

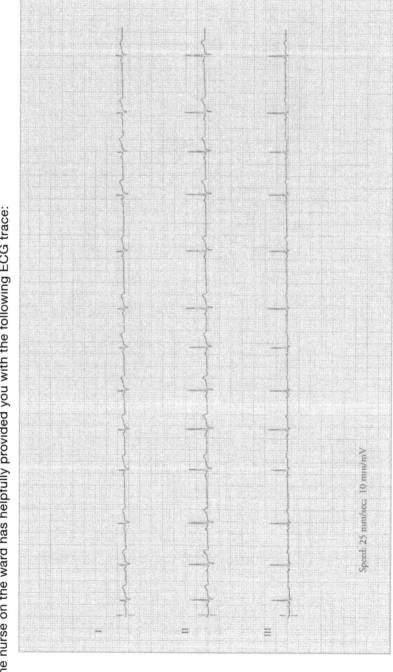

FIGURE 6.10

a Comment on the rhythm strip obtained as lead II. What is the likely significance of this finding?
b What is the likely significance of the heart murmur you have heard?
c How do you further manage this child?

Case 9

A 79-year-old scheduled for hip arthroplasty complains of intermittent dizziness and chest pain. The following ECG is obtained:

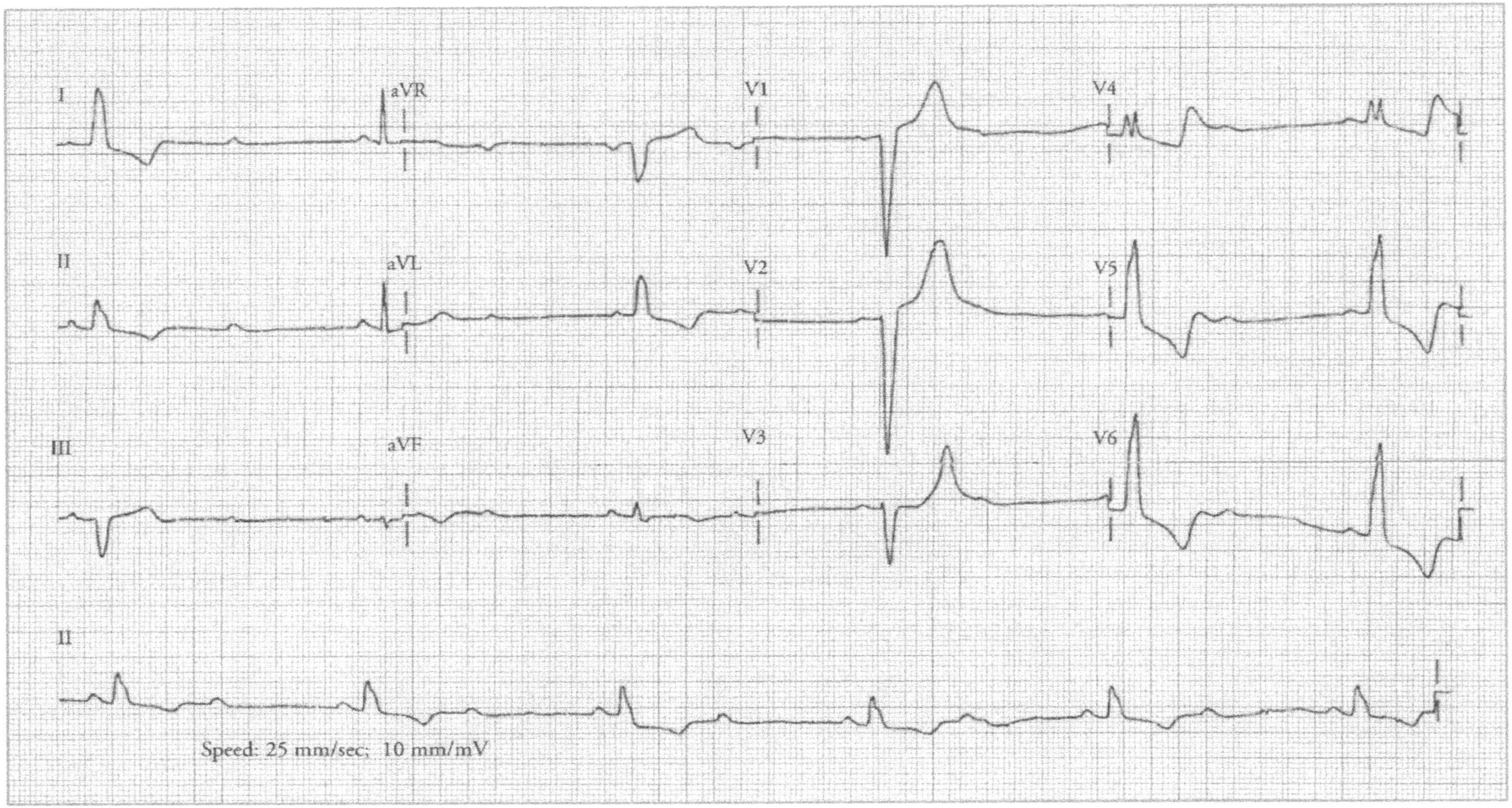

FIGURE 6.11

Speed: 25 mm/sec; 10 mm/mV

a Comment on the abnormalities present in this trace. What is your provisional diagnosis?
b What further management of the patient would you instigate before embarking on the proposed surgery?

Case 10

A 72-year-old patient complains of palpitations after undergoing carpal tunnel decompression under local anaesthesia with monitored sedation. An ECG trace is obtained as follows:

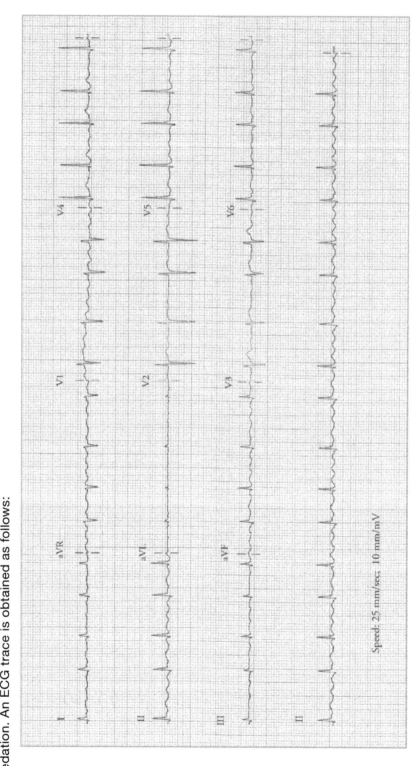

FIGURE 6.12

a Comment on this ECG. What is the diagnosis?
b How would you treat this condition?

Case 11

A 40-year-old presents with episodes of loss of consciousness of increasing frequency. One such attack occurs during admission and the following 12 lead ECG is obtained:

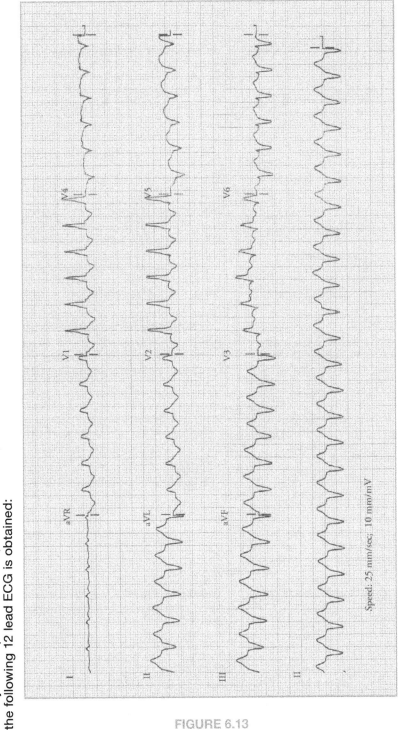

Speed: 25 mm/sec; 10 mm/mV

FIGURE 6.13

a What is your differential diagnosis?
b Describe features of this ECG that lead you to favour one provisional diagnosis.
c How would you further investigate this patient?

Case 12

A 60-year-old man with severe peripheral vascular disease complains of severe central chest pain and dyspnoea 12 hours after returning to the ward following endolumenal repair of an abdominal aortic aneurysm. This ECG was taken:

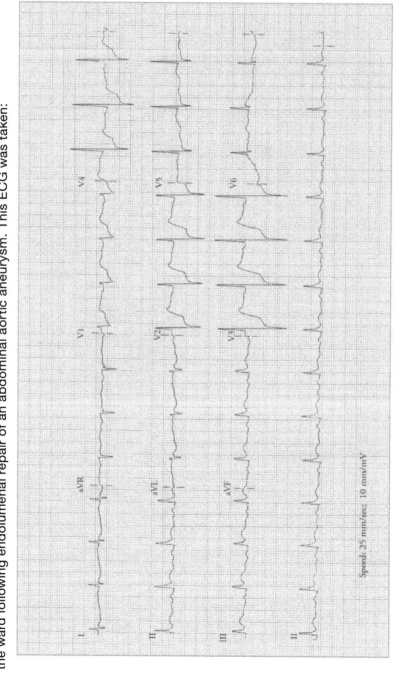

FIGURE 6.14

a What is the likely diagnosis?
b Comment on the ECG.
c Outline your further management of this gentleman.

Case 13

A 46-year-old woman is brought by ambulance to hospital with a fluctuating level of consciousness. She has had no previous admissions. She has a history of depression, for which she takes doxepin. Her other medications include cisapride for indigestion and erythromycin for a chest infection. The following ECG is obtained:

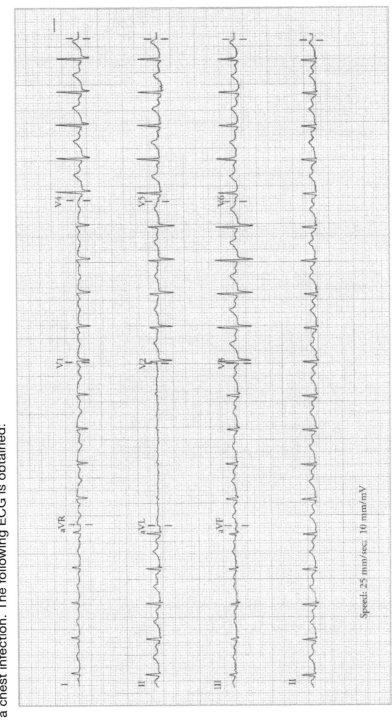

Speed: 25 mm/sec; 10 mm/mV

FIGURE 6.15

a Comment on the ECG. What is the main abnormality?

b What is the likely aetiology of this abnormality? Are there any other possible causes?

Case 14

A 39-year-old patient complains of lethargy which began one week ago and severe chest pain which began three hours ago. The following ECG is obtained:

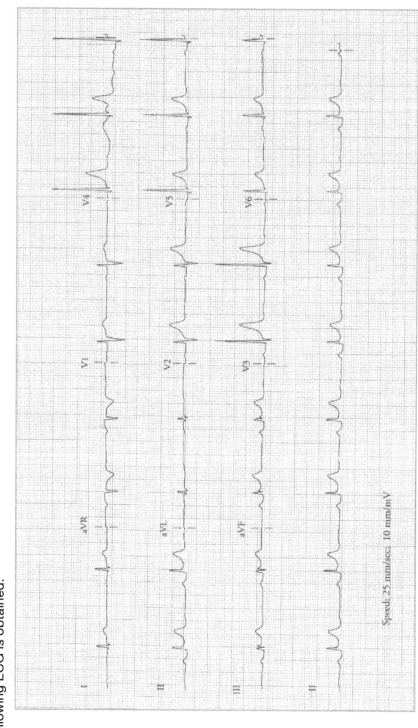

FIGURE 6.16

a Comment on the abnormalities present on the ECG. What is the likely diagnosis?

2. Chest radiography

Chest X-rays are commonly encountered, both in normal clinical practice and in the examination. While an abnormality may be immediately obvious on cursory examination, candidates should always be on the lookout for multiple abnormalities on one radiograph. To this end, it is useful to have a systematic examination checklist, as in Box 6.2.

BOX 6.2 Systematic assessment of a chest X-ray

1. Demographic and technical aspects
   - Patient ID, date and time of film.
   - Type of film (will usually have radiographical marker): postero-anterior (PA), antero-posterior (AP), lateral
     - PA film normally displaces scapulae laterally to better visualise thoracic cavity
     - Mobile and ICU films will usually be AP films
   - Position of patient: erect, supine or lateral decubitus
     - Note effects of gravity on free air and fluid
     - Significance of cardiothoracic ratio may be reduced with supine AP films
   - Adequacy of film
     - Area of interest should be completely visualised
     - Symmetric rotation: medial ends of clavicle should be equidistant from midline (vertebral spinous processes)
     - Adequate exposure: thoracic vertebrae just visible behind heart
     - Adequate inspiration: 10 posterior or 5 anterior ribs visible

2. Heart and mediastinum
   - Heart:
     - Cardiothoracic ratio on PA film should be ≤ 50%
     - Left heart border consists of left atrial appendage and left ventricle
     - Right heart border consists primarily of right atrium
     - Heart borders may be obscured by pulmonary pathology
     - Calcified or artificial heart valves may be visible
   - Trachea:
     - Should be central, moving to the right of midline due to aortic arch
     - Look for lumenal width/compression or deviation
     - Bifurcation at carina: may be widened due to mass lesion
   - Mediastinum
     - Look at shape and width of aortic arch, calcification
     - Obtain impression of overall width of mediastinum
     - Mediastinal shift: away from pneumothorax; towards collapse
     - Mediastinal air may be visible as dark shadow outlining left heart border
   - Other structures:
     - Thymus may be visible in children
     - Mediastinal lymph node enlargement at hila
     - Retrosternal goitre/other mediastinal mass
     - Tracheal/oesophageal foreign bodies
     - Pulmonary artery division into left and right branches

BOX 6.2 Systematic assessment of a chest X-ray—cont'd

3. Lungs and pleura
   - Lungs:
     - Examine for asymmetry between sides
     - Look for hyperlucency, opacification, mass lesions
     - Vascular markings generally more prominent in lower lobes and decrease towards the periphery
     - Be aware of position of fissures and lobes of each lung
     - Air bronchograms may be visible with lung consolidation
   - Pleura:
     - Thoroughly check peripheral edge of each lung for pneumothorax: lung edge visible, with hyperlucency and no lung markings lateral to this edge
     - Pleural effusions, calcifications/plaques may be visible

4. Other soft tissues
   - Diaphragm:
     - Check for clear costophrenic angles
     - Right hemidiaphragm should be higher than left
     - Subdiaphragmatic free air on erect film
     - Herniae: bubble behind heart (hiatus hernia) or bowel in chest cavity
   - Skin folds, subcutaneous emphysema, breast shadows

5. Bony structures
   - Fractures, sclerotic or lytic lesions all bones
   - Ribs: adequate inspiration, cervical rib, notching (aortic coarctation)
   - Shoulder joint, acromioclavicular joint (dislocation)

6. Indwelling devices: comment on presence and positioning
   - Endotracheal or tracheostomy tube
   - Central venous line, PICC line, pulmonary artery catheter
   - Intercostal catheter/chest drain
   - Nasogastric tube
   - Monitoring dots (ECG) and wires; pacing wires; permanent pacemakers
   - Intra-aortic balloon pump
   - Sternal wires, artificial heart valves

The following pages contain examples of some common pathologies that may be encountered on examination of chest X-rays. Note that the majority of these have a positive 'arrow sign' for ease of description; it is unlikely that candidates will be this fortunate in the examination!

The section concludes with some unlabelled examples and questions of a similar standard to those that may be expected in the clinical exam. The answers to these are on page 195.

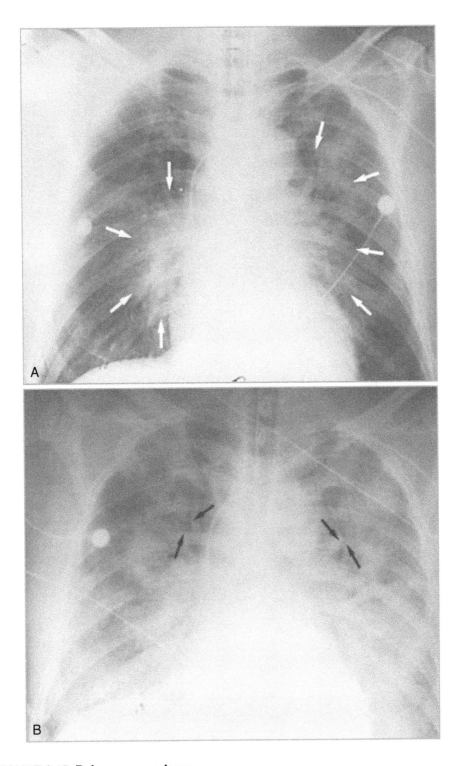

FIGURE 6.17 Pulmonary oedema

Pulmonary oedema may manifest itself as indistinctness of pulmonary vessels as they radiate from the hilum, or 'bat wing' infiltration (A). As the condition worsens (B) fluid fills the alveoli and air bronchograms (arrows) become apparent.

Source: F Mettler. Essentials of radiology. 2nd edn. Philadelphia: Elsevier Saunders, 2005.

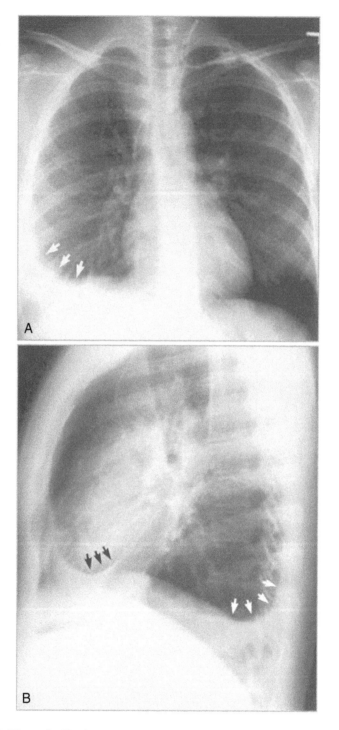

FIGURE 6.18 **Pleural effusion**
On the erect postero-anterior chest X-ray (A) there is blunting of the right costophrenic angle due to pleural fluid (arrows). The lateral view (B) shows fluid tracking into the oblique fissure (black arrows) and blunting of the posterior costophrenic angle (white arrows).

Source: F Mettler. Essentials of radiology. 2nd edn. Philadelphia: Elsevier Saunders, 2005.

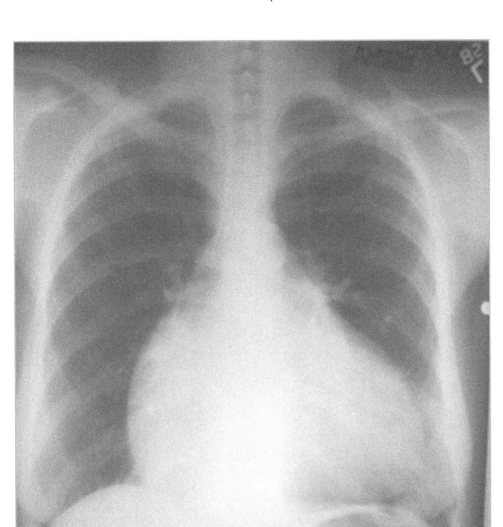

FIGURE 6.19 **Cardiomegaly**
This chest radiograph demonstrates cardiomegaly in a patient with an acute coronary syndrome. The cardiothoracic ratio is markedly increased. It is not usually possible to determine from a radiograph alone whether the increase in apparent heart size is from myocardial hypertrophy, chamber dilation or pericardial collection.
Source: J Marx, RS Hockberger, RM Walls. Rosen's emergency medicine: concepts and clinical practice. 6th edn. Elsevier Health Sciences–Mosby, 2006.

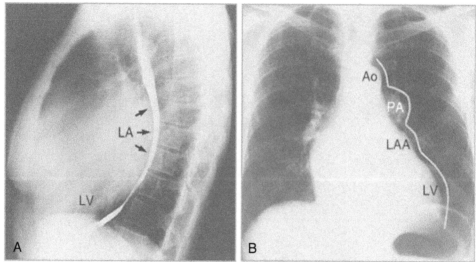

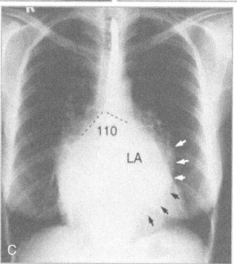

FIGURE 6.20 **Mitral stenosis**

Although mitral stenosis is becoming an increasingly uncommon clinical entity, chest radiographs of patients with the disease demonstrate some interesting features, most notably left atrial enlargement. In early stages of the disease the left atrium (LA) enlarges posteriorly and can be seen in the lateral film (A) displacing the oesophagus (filled with barium here) (arrows). As the disease progresses the left atrial appendage (LAA) may bulge out, forming a visible bulge on the postero-anterior film (B) (the so-called 'four-bump' or 'ski-mogul' sign (white outline)); the other bumps are the aorta (Ao), pulmonary artery (PA) and left ventricle (LV). Late findings in the disease are shown in film (C), and include a double-density behind the heart (arrows) and a splaying of the subcarinal angle (110° here), which normally does not exceed 75°.

Source: F Mettler. Essentials of radiology. 2nd edn. Philadelphia: Elsevier Saunders, 2005.

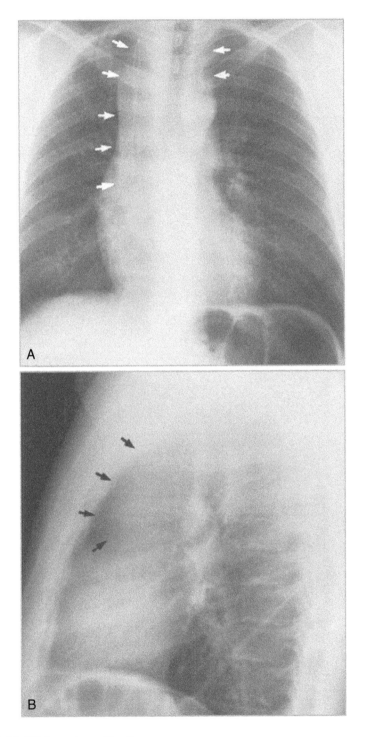

Widened mediastinum
The postero-anterior chest film (A) shows marked widening of the superior and middle mediastinum (white arrows). The lateral film (B) shows an ill-defined mass in the anterior mediastinum (black arrows), which was subsequently shown to be Hodgkin's lymphoma.
Source: F Mettler. Essentials of radiology. 2nd edn. Philadelphia: Elsevier Saunders, 2005.

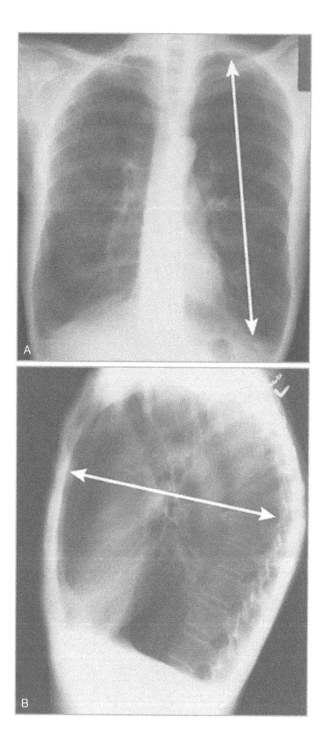

FIGURE 6.22 Emphysema
These films demonstrate emphysematous changes in chronic obstructive pulmonary disease (COPD). The postero-anterior view (A) shows that the superior aspect of the hemidiaphragms is at the same level as the posterior aspect of the twelfth ribs (arrow). Hyperinflation is also seen on the lateral view (B) as an increase in the antero-posterior diameter (arrow) and flattening of the hemidiaphragms.
Source: F Mettler. Essentials of radiology. 2nd edn. Philadelphia: Elsevier Saunders, 2005.

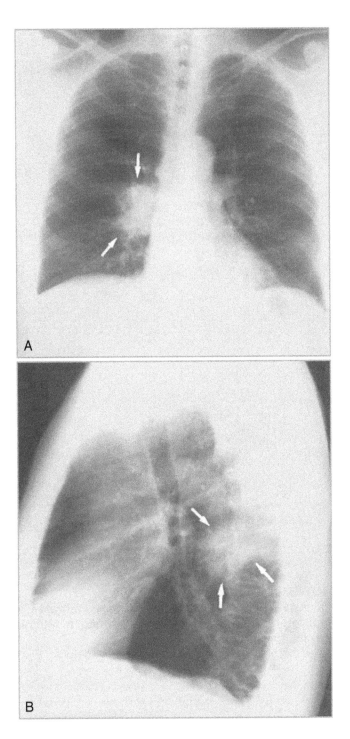

FIGURE 6.23 Pulmonary mass
An ill-defined mass is noted on the postero-anterior chest X-ray (arrows) (A).
Although this appears to be located near the right hilum, the lateral chest X-ray
(B) clearly shows the mass to be posterior to the hilum. Its shaggy appearance
is very suggestive of carcinoma.
Source: F Mettler. Essentials of radiology. 2nd edn. Philadelphia: Elsevier Saunders,
2005.

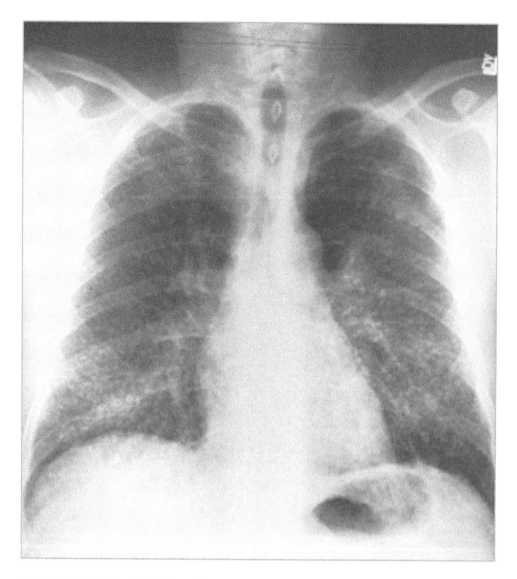

FIGURE 6.24 **Interstitial lung disease**
In this X-ray of a patient with sarcoidosis, diffuse infiltrates are present in
the parenchymal interstitium of both lungs, forming a reticular shadowing
predominantly in the lower zones.
Source: F Mettler. Essentials of radiology. 2nd edn. Philadelphia: Elsevier Saunders, 2005.

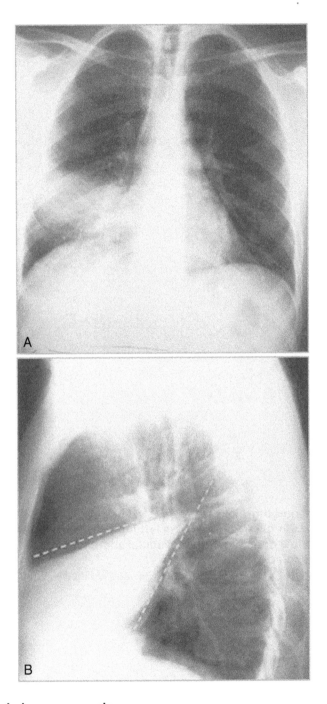

FIGURE 6.25 **Lobar pneumonia**
Right middle lobe pneumonia. On the postero-anterior chest X-ray (A), the alveolar infiltrate obscures the right cardiac border. This silhouette sign means that the pathologic process is up against the right cardiac border and therefore must be in the middle lobe. This is confirmed on the lateral view (B) by noting that the consolidation is anterior to the oblique fissure but below the horizontal fissure (dashed lines).
Source: F Mettler. Essentials of radiology. 2nd edn. Philadelphia: Elsevier Saunders, 2005.

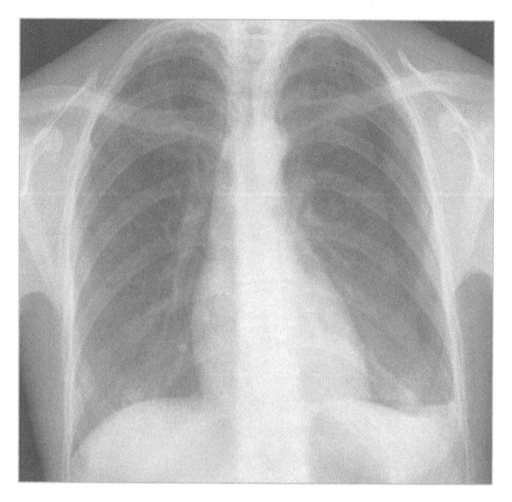

FIGURE 6.26 **Pneumothorax**

Chest X-ray taken in full expiration. The left lung has partially collapsed and an area of extreme low density without vascular markings is visible peripheral to a well-defined lung edge.

Source: A Adam, AK Dixon (eds). Grainger and Allison's diagnostic radiology. 5th edn. Elsevier Churchill Livingstone, 2008.

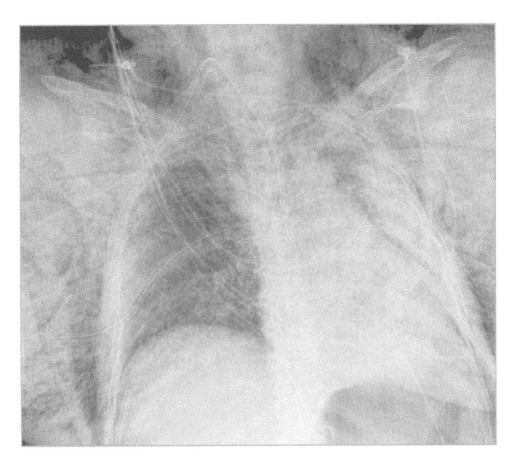

FIGURE 6.27 **Airway trauma**

This patient sustained partial tracheal transection in a motorbike accident. An oral RAE endotracheal tube was inserted at the scene, and can be seen in situ. Pneumomediastinum is present. Bilateral multiple rib fractures with pulmonary contusion were also sustained, and chest tubes are present bilaterally. Extensive subcutaneous emphysema can be seen in the soft tissues of the chest wall and neck.

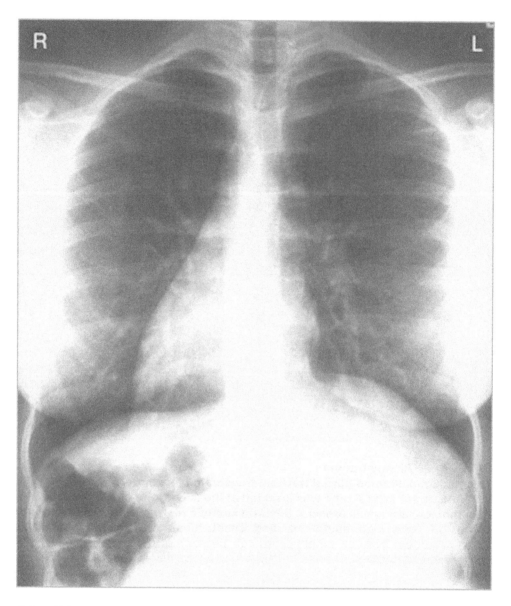

FIGURE 6.28
Source: F Mettler. Essentials of radiology. 2nd edn. Philadelphia: Elsevier Saunders, 2005.

Case 15
A 60-year-old woman has the above chest X-ray taken during routine screening prior to knee arthroplasty:
a What is the diagnosis?
b What other investigations do you require?

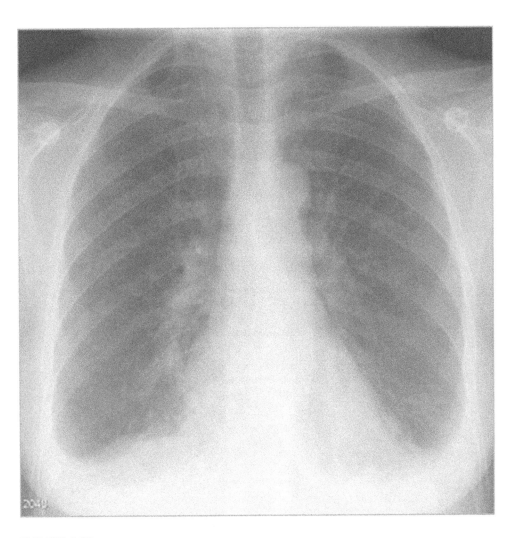

FIGURE 6.29
Source: A Adam, AK Dixon (eds). Grainger and Allison's diagnostic radiology, 5th edn.
Elsevier Churchill Livingstone, 2008.

Case 16

A 48-year-old woman with known ovarian carcinoma presents with shortness of breath at rest. The above erect postero-anterior chest X-ray is taken:

a Is there any abnormality on this film which might account for the patient's symptoms?

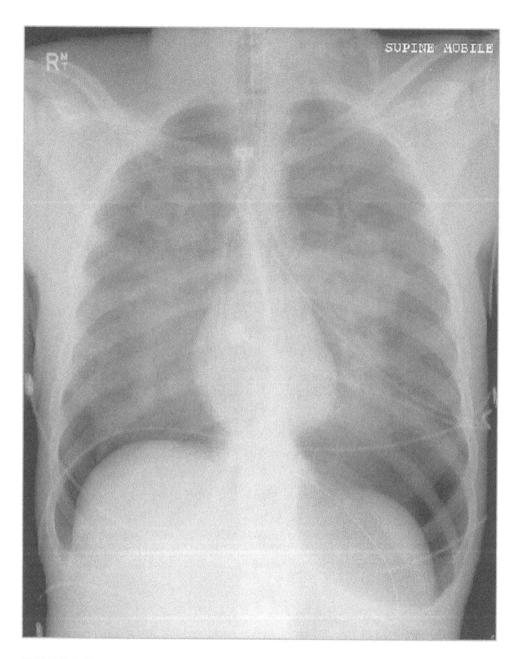

FIGURE 6.30

Case 17

A 30-year-old asthmatic man requires ongoing intubation and mechanical ventilation after severe bronchospasm diagnosed during surgery for laparoscopic hernia repair. The above chest X-ray is taken on day 2 of his admission:

a Describe the medical devices apparent on this X-ray.
b Is there any pathological abnormality which might account for ongoing hypoxia in this man?

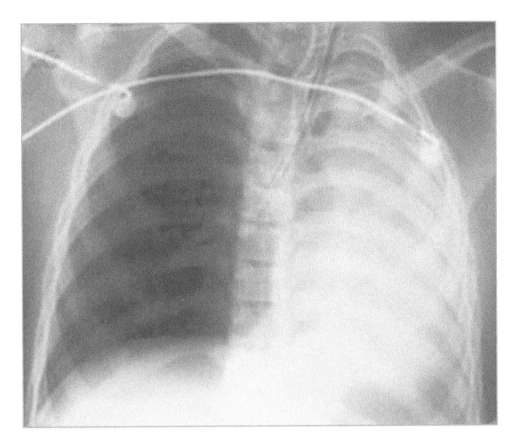

FIGURE 6.31
Source: F Mettler. Essentials of radiology. 2nd edn. Philadelphia: Elsevier Saunders, 2005.

Case 18

An otherwise well 14-year-old boy becomes increasingly hypoxic during left tympanoplasty surgery. The above portable film is taken at the end of the case:
a Describe the abnormalities on this film.
b What clinical signs would you expect to elicit in this patient?

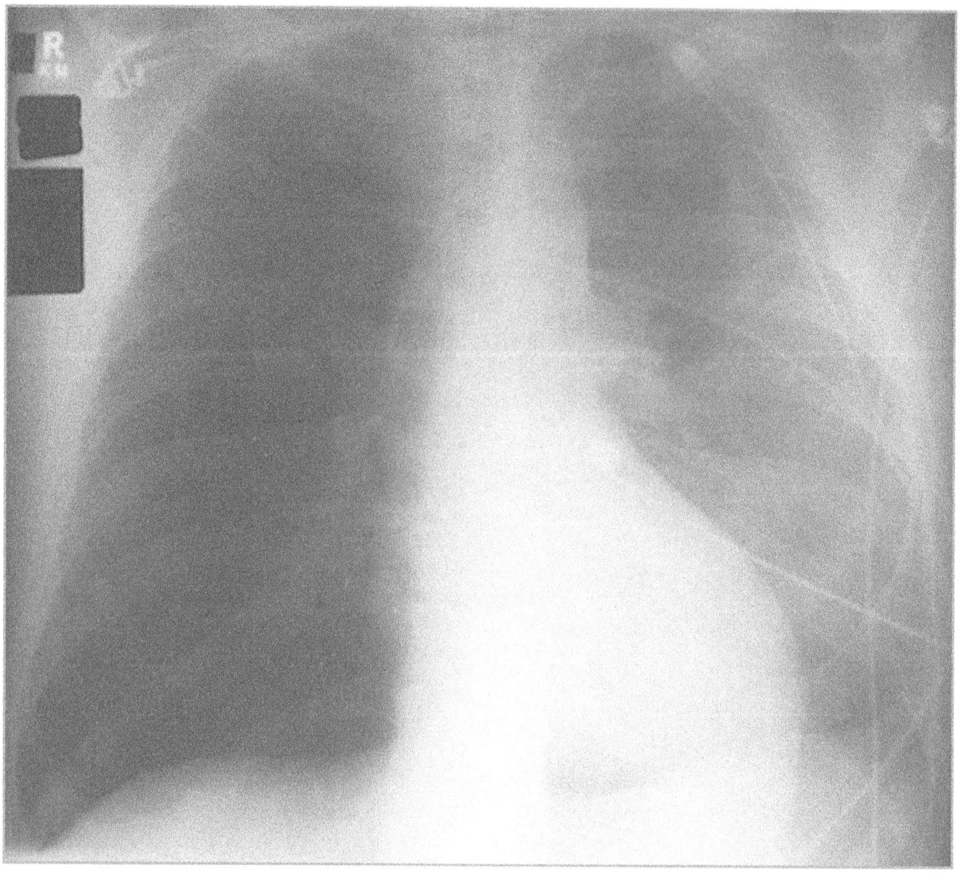

FIGURE 6.32
Source: A Adam, AK Dixon (eds). Grainger and Allison's diagnostic radiology. 5th edn. Elsevier Churchill Livingstone, 2008.

Case 19
A 24-year-old man sustained severe injuries in a motor vehicle accident and returns to your rural intensive care unit following a laparotomy and splenectomy. The above routine chest film is taken the next morning:
a Describe this chest X-ray and any abnormalities that may be present.

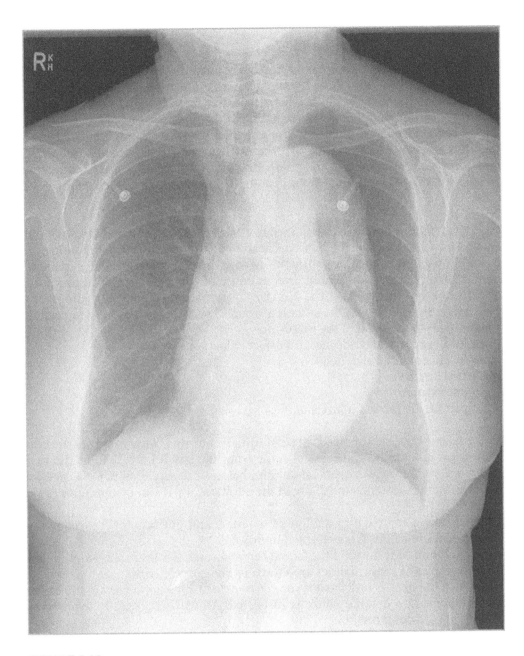

FIGURE 6.33

Case 20

A 55-year-old woman presents with shortness of breath 3 weeks after laparoscopic cholecystectomy. She is a heavy smoker. Her postero-anterior chest radiograph appears above:

a Describe the abnormalities present on this film.

b What other investigations do you require?

3. Neck radiography

The cervical spine is of particular interest to the anaesthetist because of conditions that may imperil the spinal cord with airway manipulation. For this reason you are expected to know how and in what circumstances to image the cervical spine, and to be reasonably adept at interpretation of the films.

The classic scenarios that may present themselves to the anaesthetist (and therefore the exam candidate) are the patient with neck trauma requiring operation for other injuries and the patient with rheumatoid arthritis or (less frequently) Down syndrome who may suffer from atlanto-axial subluxation.

Neck trauma

A cervical spine injury must be assumed in a patient who has suffered a major blunt trauma until the spine can be cleared. Clearance involves clinical and radiological examination, and cannot be satisfactorily completed if there is either a painful, distracting injury or a decreased level of consciousness, be it from head injury, intoxication or other causes. The NEXUS (National Emergency X-Radiography Utilization Study) defined the situation where a neck X-ray was *not* required in trauma. This includes all of the following:

- no midline cervical tenderness on direct palpation
- no focal neurological deficit
- normal alertness
- no intoxication
- no painful distracting injuries.

The lateral cervical film needs to be of sufficient quality. Always ensure the film allows you to visualise the cervical spine from the base of the skull to the first thoracic vertebra. An adequate lateral film has a sensitivity of 85% for a cervical fracture, and this extends to 92% with the addition of AP and open mouth (peg) views.

A systematic approach to the film is required, and one scheme for evaluating the cervical spine film(s) is presented in Box 6.3.

Key anatomical features of the lateral cervical spine X-ray are shown in Figure 6.34. Examples of abnormalities are shown in Figures 6.35–6.38.

A CT of the neck is indicated if you are unable to get a good view of the entire cervical spine or a definite injury is suspected. An MRI is generally required to evaluate a cord compression.

BOX 6.3 Systematic assessment of neck radiographs

1. Demographic and technical aspects
   - Patient ID, date
   - Type of film
     - AP, lateral, peg views

2. Alignment
   - Symmetry on AP film
   - Anterior and posterior vertebral lines
   - Spinous processes
   - Spinolaminal line

3. Bony deformity
   - Cervicocranium
     - Anterior and posterior arch of C1
     - Odontoid peg, body of C2
     - Atlantodental space
   - Lower cervical vertebrae
     - Fracture or compression of vertebral body
     - Fracture of spinous process

4. Spinal canal
   - Space narrowing

5. Prevertebral soft tissues
   - Abnormal thickening indicating soft tissue swelling

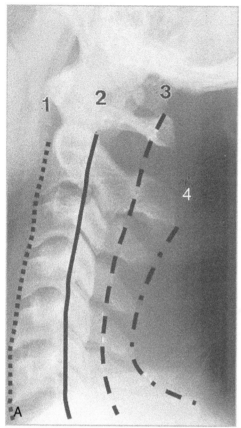
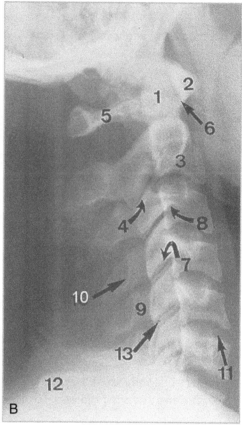

FIGURE 6.34 Lateral cervical spine
(A) Normal alignment of the cervical vertebrae:
1. Anterior vertebral line
2. Posterior vertebral line
3. Spinolaminal line
4. Spinous processes

(B) Key anatomical features:
1. Odontoid peg
2. Anterior arch of C1
3. C2 body
4. Superior articular process
5. Posterior arch of C1
6. Atlanto-odontal space
7. Inferior articular process
8. Pedicle
9. Lamina
10. Base of spinous process
11. Disc
12. Spinous process
13. C5–C6 joint

Source: N Blackwell, C Foot, C Thomas. Examination intensive care and anaesthesia. Elsevier, 2007.

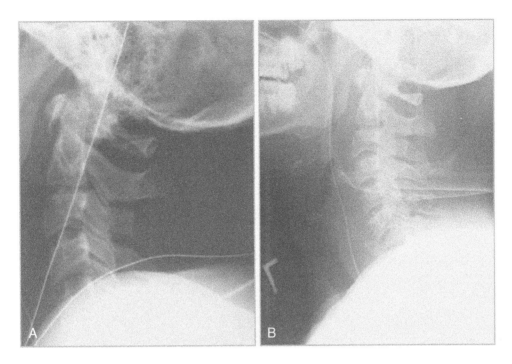

FIGURE 6.35 **Burst fracture of C7**
The importance of completely visualising all seven cervical vertebrae.
(A) Inadequate cross-table lateral cervical spine radiograph (C7 not visualised).
(B) A repeat lateral film on the right demonstrates a burst fracture of C7.
Source: CM Townsend, RD Beauchamp, BM Evers, KL Mattox. Sabiston textbook of surgery. 18th edn. Philadelphia: Elsevier Saunders, 2007.

FIGURE 6.36 **Fracture–dislocation**
Fracture–dislocation at C4–5. There is a disruption of the facet joints and the intervertebral disc with characteristic anterior displacement of the vertebra above the level of the dislocation. The interspinous ligaments are also disrupted, as evidenced by the separation of the spinous processes.
Source: A Adam, AK Dixon (eds). Grainger and Allison's diagnostic radiology. 5th edn. Elsevier Churchill Livingstone, 2008.

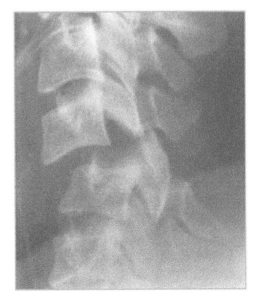

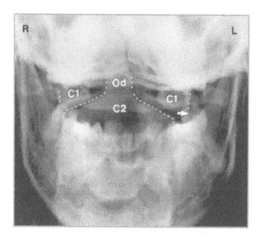

FIGURE 6.37 Jefferson fracture
Burst fracture of C1. On this open-mouth antero-posterior view, widening of the space between the odontoid and the left lateral mass of C1 is apparent. The lateral aspect also projects past the lateral margin of C2 (arrow).
Source: F Mettler. Essentials of radiology. 2nd edn. Philadelphia: Elsevier Saunders, 2005.

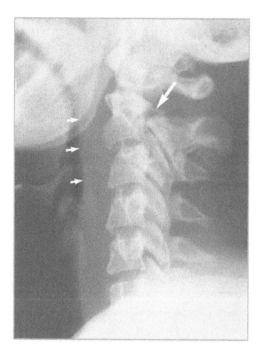

FIGURE 6.38 Hangman's fracture
The lateral view of the cervical spine demonstrates marked soft tissue swelling anterior to C1, C2 and C3 (small white arrows). A fracture line is seen just posterior to the body of C2 (large arrow).
Source: F Mettler. Essentials of radiology. 2nd edn. Philadelphia: Elsevier Saunders, 2005.

Flexion/extension views

About 25% of patients with rheumatoid arthritis develop a degree of atlanto-axial subluxation. In most cases this is due to the destruction of the transverse ligament, and leads to anterior subluxation where the C1 vertebra moves forward relative to C2 and risks spinal cord compression by the odontoid peg. This effect is accentuated by neck flexion, and subluxation is deemed to exist when there is a >4 mm (>3 mm in younger patients) distance between the atlas and the odontoid peg (Fig 6.39). Posterior subluxation is due to the destruction of the odontoid peg and is accentuated with the neck in flexion. Preoperative neck imaging is required if the patient complains of neck or neurological symptoms.

About 30% of patients with Down syndrome suffer from atlanto-axial instability, probably as a result of congenital laxity of the transverse ligament. Routine cervical spine views are generally considered unnecessary.

Patients with ankylosing spondylosis also rarely develop atlanto-axial subluxation, but the principal airway concern is the progressive ankylosis and kyphosis, making direct laryngoscopy difficult, and at the risk of trauma to the neck. Assessment is essentially clinical and neck X-rays are not usually ordered preoperatively.

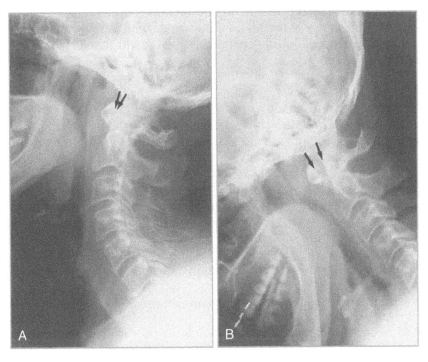

FIGURE 6.39 Flexion/extension views in rheumatoid arthritis
Instability of the transverse ligament of C1 in rheumatoid arthritis. A lateral view of the cervical spine with the neck extended (A) shows very little space (which is normal) between the posterior aspect of the arch of C1 and the anterior portion of the odontoid (arrows). With flexion (B), this space markedly widens, and the odontoid is free to compress the spinal cord, which is posterior to it.
Source: F Mettler. Essentials of radiology. 2nd edn. Philadelphia: Elsevier Saunders, 2005.

4. Computed tomography (CT)

Computed tomography is an imaging modality commonly employed in many fields of medicine. It is of importance for the anaesthetist as a tool for rapid assessment of the trauma patient, and is the gold standard in the diagnosis of many intracranial, intrathoracic and intra-abdominal conditions with implications for anaesthesia.

CT scanning is performed by taking a large number of two-dimensional X-ray images around a single axis of rotation, achieved by passing a rotating fan of X-rays through the area of interest and measuring the transmission at thousands of points. Early scanners rotated an X-ray tube once around the patient to take a single 'slice' of information, then the gantry was moved further into the scanner to take the next slice and so on. Newer scanners continuously rotate, irradiate the patient and measure data as the table moves (hence the terms spiral or helical scanning), often with multiple rows of detectors, allowing much faster and more accurate scans. Transmission data is stored and processed on powerful computers. In addition to displaying series of two-dimensional axial slices, modern CT scanners are capable of displaying images in other reformatted planes of the body, or even in three dimensions. The orientation for viewing axial slices is as if you were looking at the patient from the foot of the bed (i.e. the left side of the film is the right side of the patient, and the top of the film is usually the anterior part of the patient). Appearance of tissues on CT scans depends largely on the computer manipulation employed, but in general air is black, soft tissue is grey, and bone and contrast agents are white.

Head and neck CT

CT scanning is the investigation of choice in major head trauma and suspected haemorrhagic stroke. While lacking the degree of soft-tissue definition afforded by magnetic resonance imaging, CT scanning is quicker, more accessible and safer in the acute setting, as well as providing better bone imaging. Anaesthetic management of the mechanically ventilated patient is considerably easier in the CT scanner than in the MRI suite.

Many algorithms exist for diagnostic imaging in acute spinal injury. In general, CT scanning is useful when definitive signs of an injury are present, when the patient is neurologically obtunded or when plain X-rays are inadequate for visualising the entire cervical spine. CT scanning is also helpful in evaluating soft tissue involvement in other conditions such as neck abscess or thyroid enlargement.

Some examples of head and neck CT scans are provided in Figures 6.40–6.44.

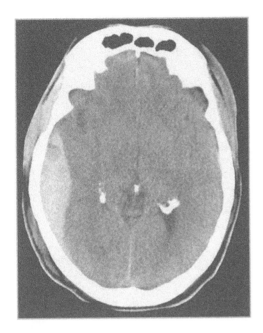

FIGURE 6.40 **Extradural haematoma**
There is a large biconvex right temporal
extradural collection containing a small
round lucency caused by active fresh
bleeding from the middle meningeal
artery. There is also some midline shift
and ventricular effacement.
Source: A Adam, AK Dixon (eds). Grainger and Allison's diagnostic radiology. 5th edn. Elsevier Churchill Livingstone, 2008.

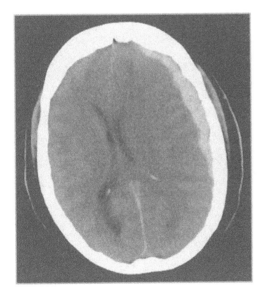

FIGURE 6.41 **Acute subdural**
haematoma
This film shows an irregular hetero-
geneous density overlying the left
cerebral cortex, with marked midline
shift and ventricular effacement.
Source: A Adam, AK Dixon (eds). Grainger and Allison's diagnostic radiology. 5th edn. Elsevier Churchill Livingstone, 2008.

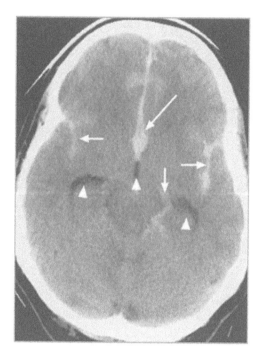

FIGURE 6.42 **Subarachnoid haemorrhage**
This scan shows diffuse subarachnoid blood (short arrows) and a haematoma in the septum pellucidum indicating that the likely source is an aneurysm of the anterior communicating artery (long diagonal arrow). The temporal horns of the lateral ventricles and anterior recess of the third ventricle are enlarged (triangle arrowheads) due to secondary communicating hydrocephalus.
Source: A Adam, AK Dixon (eds). Grainger and Allison's diagnostic radiology. 5th edn. Elsevier Churchill Livingstone, 2008.

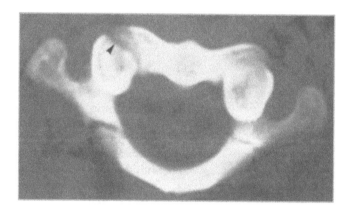

FIGURE 6.43 **Jefferson fracture of Atlas**
This CT demonstrates a single fracture in the right portion of the anterior arch (arrowhead) and bilateral fractures of the posterior arch of C1.
Source: A Adam, AK Dixon (eds). Grainger and Allison's diagnostic radiology. 5th edn. Elsevier Churchill Livingstone, 2008.

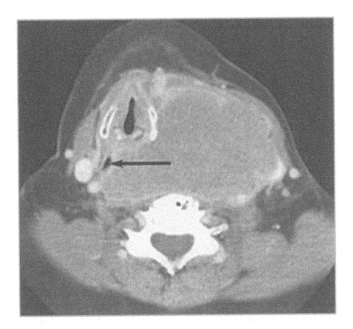

FIGURE 6.44 Thyroid goitre with airway displacement
This contrast-enhanced axial CT slice was taken at the level of the larynx. The
left thyroid gland is replaced by a large mass which displaces the larynx and
oesophagus (black arrow).
Source: CW Cummings (ed.). Otolaryngology: head and neck surgery. 4th edn. Elsevier
Mosby, 2005.

Chest CT

Acute indications for CT scanning of the chest include CT pulmonary angiography
for suspected pulmonary thromboembolism, chest trauma and evaluation of
acute aortic syndromes (e.g. dissection). In the non-acute setting CT scanning
is commonly used for evaluation of mediastinal masses present on plain films,
characterising interstitial lung disease, detecting pulmonary metastases and
identifying small airway disease or bronchiectasis. Other pathologies may, of
course, also be detected on CT scans, as illustrated in Figures 6.45–6.48.

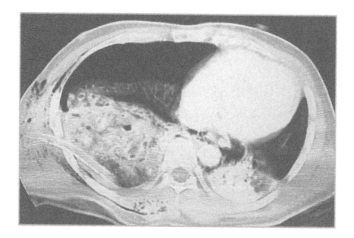

FIGURE 6.45 **Tension pneumothorax**
This CT image demonstrates a post-traumatic pneumothorax. Rib fracture is evident on the right side. Despite the presence of an intercostal drain a tension pneumothorax was developing as the drain was blocked with congealed blood. The right-sided pneumothorax is situated anteriorly and the mediastinum is displaced to the left due to the tension.
Source: A Adam, AK Dixon (eds). Grainger and Allison's diagnostic radiology. 5th edn. Elsevier Churchill Livingstone, 2008.

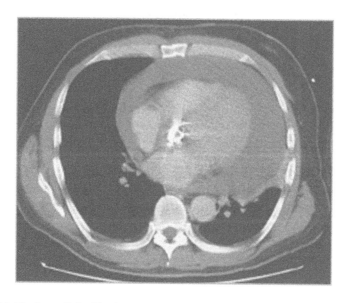

FIGURE 6.46 **Pericardial effusion**
This film is from a patient who had demonstrated cardiomegaly on a plain X-ray after aortic valve replacement surgery. Unenhanced CT through the level of the valve replacement demonstrates a large pericardial effusion.
Source: A Adam, AK Dixon (eds). Grainger and Allison's diagnostic radiology. 5th edn. Elsevier Churchill Livingstone, 2008.

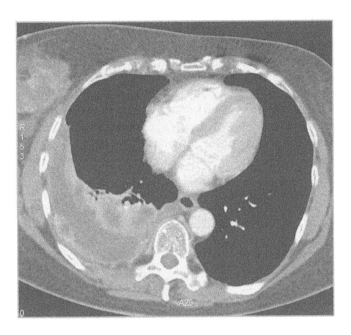

FIGURE 6.47 **Malignant pleural effusion**
In this right pleural effusion, CT identifies the extensive and irregular pleural thickening characteristic of a malignant process (pleural metastases). Note also the primary tumour in the right breast.
Source: A Adam, AK Dixon (eds). Grainger and Allison's diagnostic radiology. 5th edn. Elsevier Churchill Livingstone, 2008.

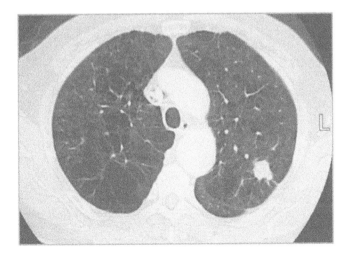

FIGURE 6.48 **Emphysema**
CT image from a patient with upper zone predominant emphysema showing thickened septae and widespread airspace destruction. The mass in the left upper lobe is a probable lung cancer.
Source: A Adam, AK Dixon (eds). Grainger and Allison's diagnostic radiology. 5th edn. Elsevier Churchill Livingstone, 2008.

Abdominal CT

Computed tomography is extremely useful for imaging solid abdominal viscera, peritoneum and retroperitoneal structures. The entire abdomen and pelvis can be imaged in less than 10 minutes. Scans can be taken after ingestion of oral contrast (which helps differentiate bowel from other soft tissues) and intravenous contrast (for visualisation of vascular structures, kidneys, ureter and bladder). Rectal contrast can also be given if pelvic pathology is suspected. Examples of abdominal CT scans are shown in Figures 6.49 and 6.50.

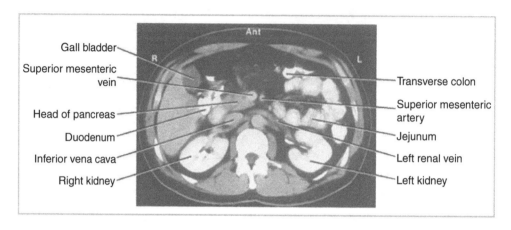

FIGURE 6.49 Abdominal CT
CT scan of abdomen at level of L1. The patient had received intravenous and oral contrast.
Source: F Mettler. Essentials of radiology. 2nd edn. Philadelphia: Elsevier Saunders, 2005.

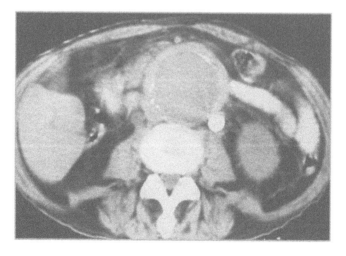

FIGURE 6.50 Abdominal aortic aneurysm
Contrast-enhanced CT demonstrates a significant sized abdominal aortic aneurysm with a thick, well-defined outer wall. There is hydroureter on the left and hydroureter with a non-functioning kidney on the right. These features are typical of inflammatory abdominal aortic aneurysm.
Source: A Adam, AK Dixon (eds). Grainger and Allison's diagnostic radiology. 5th edn. Elsevier Churchill Livingstone, 2008.

5. Magnetic resonance imaging (MRI)

The MRI scanner holds interest for the anaesthetist for two specific reasons:
- We are required to anaesthetise children and the occasional adult who is unable to remain still in the scanner in order to obtain satisfactory images.
- The MRI remains the imaging modality of choice for the emergency investigation of prolonged block following central neuraxial blockade, specifically looking for haemorrhage or epidural abscess.

The principal advantages of imaging with MRI over CT scanning are its better soft tissue differentiation. Bone also produces minimal signal, therefore neural structures that are surrounded by bone (such as spinal cord and the posterior cranial fossa) are imaged with greater clarity. There is also no risk from ionising radiation.

Basic physics

Atomic nuclei with an odd number of protons or neutrons have a potential to act as magnetic dipoles due to the nature of their 'spin'. Although this can be a feature of all paramagnetic elements, hydrogen (with its single proton) is the element of interest for standard MR imaging.

The patient is placed in a powerful superconductor electromagnet (cooled with liquid helium at about 4 Kelvin) with field strength of up to 3.0 T (Tesla). This is produced by the large coil that surrounds the patient, i.e. the tunnel. The hydrogen nuclei align their magnetic spin with the field and can subsequently be flipped in and out of alignment by high frequency magnetic pulses that are applied at right angles to the main field. As the nuclei flip back into alignment they produce minute radio frequency signals, which are detected and form the basis of the image.

The problems with anaesthesia for MRI scanning relate to the difficult access to the patient, physical dangers relating to the magnetic field (which is always on), current induction caused by the magnet, noise, and electrical interference degrading the image quality. Detailed discussion regarding anaesthesia for MRI falls outside the scope of this book.

Types of magnetic resonance image

The hydrogen nucleus (proton) is switched perpendicular to the main field by the additional magnetic field. Once the transverse magnetic pulse is turned off, the longitudinal magnetisation recovers exponentially with a time constant of T1 (called longitudinal or T1 relaxation). The loss of phase coherence in the transverse plane is called the transverse or T2 relaxation. These times are around 1 second for the T1 and an order of magnitude faster for the T2 relaxation. These values vary widely between tissues, which allows good tissue differentiation of MRI.

The practical difference between the two types of scan is that the T1-weighted scan has water displayed as dark and the T2 has water displayed as bright. If you are presented with a head or spinal cord scan, a quick look at the CSF will allow you to easily differentiate them and avoid an interpretative error. Pathology such as oedema fluid will show up as a bright halo on the T2-weighted scan.

Contrast agents used in MRI are typically gadolinium compounds. The contrast is paramagnetic and decreases the relaxation time constant of the tissue being imaged. The effect of the gadolinium is to make enhanced tissue bright on the T1 weighted image, which is useful for the detection of vascular tumours and in the assessment of tissue perfusion.

In addition to these basic types of image, MRI scanners are able to produce a range of sophisticated image types including angiography, spectroscopy, diffusion MRI and others. Of these, the use of MRI angiography for the imaging of the coronary arteries may well become important to the anaesthetist as the technology improves.

The accompanying MRI examples illustrate differences between T1 and T2 weighted scans, and show some examples of spinal pathology (Figs 6.51–6.54).

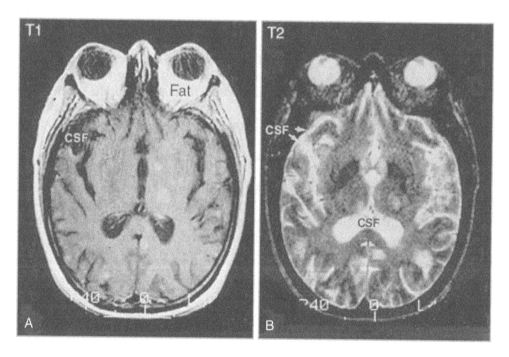

FIGURE 6.51 **T1- and T2-weighted scans: head**
Magnetic resonance (MR) imaging of the brain. Film (A) shows T1 images in which fat appears white, water or cerebrospinal fluid (CSF) appears black, and brain and muscle appear grey. In almost all MR images bone gives off no signal and will appear black. With T2 imaging (B), fat is dark, and water and CSF have a high signal and will appear bright or white. The brain and soft tissues still appear grey.
Source: F Mettler. Essentials of radiology. 2nd edn. Philadelphia: Elsevier Saunders, 2005.

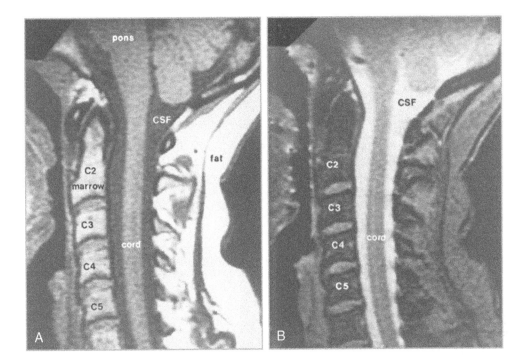

FIGURE 6.52 T1- andT2-weighted scans: cervical spine
Normal appearance of the cervical spine and spinal cord on magnetic resonance imaging. A sagittal (lateral) view with a T1-weighted sequence (A) shows that the subcutaneous fat and marrow within the vertebral bodies have a high signal and appear white.The cerebrospinal fluid (CSF) appears almost black, and the cerebellum, pons and spinal cord appear grey. On the T2-weighted sequence (B) the contrast is somewhat reversed, with fluid or CSF appearing white and the fat becoming dark.The spinal cord remains grey.
Source: F Mettler. Essentials of radiology. 2nd edn. Philadelphia: Elsevier Saunders, 2005.

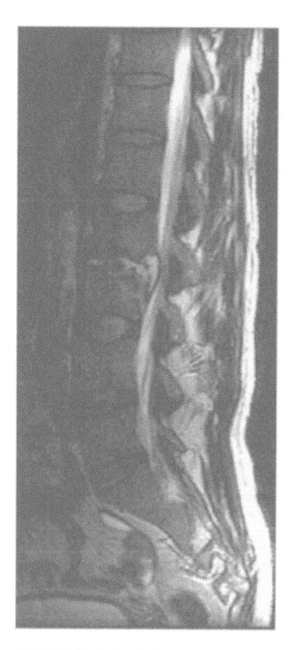

FIGURE 6.53 **Epidural abscess**
T2-weighted scan of the lumbosacral spine showing a lesion in the anterior epidural space compressing the thecal sac posteriorly. There is associated discitis of the L2–3 disc.
Source: L Goldman. Cecil medicine. 23rd edn. Elsevier Saunders, 2007.

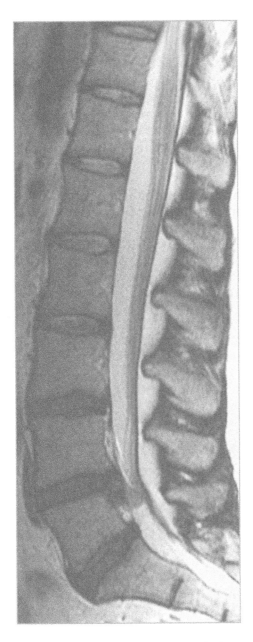

FIGURE 6.54 **Lumbar disc herniation**
Midline sagittal T2-weighted MRI of the lumbar spine with good demonstration of conus (normal) and cauda equina. The intervertebral discs down to L2/3 are relatively normal with degenerate discs between L3 and S1. At L4/5 there is extensive herniation of disc material, which is migrating caudally and extending posteriorly through the posterior longitudinal ligament.
Source: A Adam, AK Dixon (eds). Grainger and Allison's diagnostic radiology. 5th edn. Elsevier Churchill Livingstone, 2008.

6. Echocardiography

Echocardiography is unique in its ability to provide detailed structural and functional information about the heart and major vessels non-invasively. As the technology improves and access becomes easier, a larger proportion of patients are having an echocardiograph as part of their perioperative management. Coupled with this, an increasing number of anaesthetists (examiners included) are becoming competent in echocardiography. This means that the candidate presenting for the final FANZCA exam should have a reasonable understanding of the modality.

Candidates should have had some exposure to intraoperative transoesophageal echocardiography (TOE) during the course of their cardiothoracic module. Although TOE has distinct advantages in terms of image resolution, especially of posteriorly located structures, the assessment of ventricular function and valve gradients is often less accurate. This, coupled with its relatively invasive nature and the requirement for sedation, means that the vast majority of echo reports relating to the perioperative patient will be the result of a transthoracic examination.

Apart from its obvious advantage in the intraoperative setting, TOE is specifically indicated in a number of situations. These include:
- assessment of the mitral valve prior to surgery
- assessment of prosthetic valve function
- diagnosis of endocarditis and assessment of its complications
- detection of thrombus in the left atrial appendage
- diagnosis of aortic dissection
- detection of suspected cardiac masses.

It may also be indicated in situations where a transthoracic study is unable to provide useful information, such as the unstable, ventilated postcardiac surgical patient.

It is clearly not (yet) expected that the candidate would be able to interpret echocardiography images. Indeed, the capacity to show echo loops in the exam situation is not available. However, the candidate should expect to be handed an echo report and be able to interpret the information and relate it to a patient or clinical scenario.

How to interpret the report

The standard transthoracic examination will use four modalities to examine the heart:
1. M-mode (motion mode), a one-dimensional representation of movement versus time. Generally it is used to measure the size and movement of the aorta, left atrium and left ventricle.
2. Two-dimensional real-time images (the moving pictures of the heart).
3. Spectral Doppler, which measures the velocity of blood flow.
4. Colour flow Doppler, which shows blood flow as a colour map superimposed on a moving two-dimensional image.

Information from all these modalities is incorporated in the standard echocardiography report.

By far the most time efficient and useful expedient in the exam situation is to head straight to the summary of findings, if it is present. You may be asked to comment on these findings and relate the significance to anaesthesia. In some situations you may be asked to pass comment on the main part of the report, which at first glance can be a bewildering collection of numbers and abbreviations.

Which numbers matter and what do they mean?

In many reports a significant number of the parameters are not recorded. This may be due to the fact that the structure was clearly normal (why record the gradient across a normal valve?), or the image quality was poor. Assume in the exam that if the value is not there it is not significant. The components of a representative patient report are outlined in Tables 6.1–6.5.

M-mode measurement

TABLE 6.1 M-mode measurements					
LVIDd	4.5 cm	Left atrium	4.0 cm	LV mass	gm
LVIDs	3.0 cm	Aortic root	2.8 cm	LV mass (corrected)	gm
IVS	1.3 cm	LA:Ao ratio	1.4	Dia vol	mL
Posterior wall	1.3 cm	Right ventricle	cm	Sys vol	mL
FS	33 %	SV	56 mL	EF	61 %
ProxAscAorta:	cm				

This represents the one-dimensional measurements of the heart. The internal diameter of the left ventricle is expressed in diastole and systole (4.5–3.0 cm in this case), and the percentage change is represented as the fractional shortening (FS, 33%). There is an ejection fraction (EF) calculated from the FS. The normal range for the diastolic diameter of the left ventricle (LVIDd) is quite large and depends on the size of the patient, but if it is greater than about 5.5 cm then LV dilatation is probably present.

The diastolic thickness of the septum and posterior wall are present (1.3 cm each). The upper limit of normal is 1.1 cm for females and 1.2 cm for males. Therefore, this patient has LV hypertrophy. The upper limit of normal for the left atrium is about 4.5 cm.

Aortic valve Doppler haemodynamics

TABLE 6.2 Doppler haemodynamics: Aortic valve					
V2 (Vmax)	1.9 m/sec	Peak gradient	14 mmHg	Aortic V2 VTI	29 cm
Mean gradient	6 mmHg	AVAmax	1.8 cm²	AVA VTI	1.8 cm²
LVOT diameter	2.0 cm	LVOT (VTI)	16.0 cm	Regurgitation	trivial
AR pt1/2	ms	AI slope	m/sec²	Stenosis	

This section of the report is compiled by measuring the physical dimensions of the left ventricular outflow tract (LVOT) and the blood flow patterns through the LVOT and the aortic valve. The important numbers are the area of the aortic valve (AVA), which is 1.8 cm² and the mean gradient (6 mmHg). The interpretation of these is given in Table 6.6 on page 160. The degree of regurgitation should be recorded if it is significant.

Mitral valve Doppler haemodynamics

TABLE 6.3 Doppler haemodynamics: Mitral valve

E wave	0.9 m/sec	A wave	0.6 m/sec	E:A ratio	1.7
A wave duration	ms	Decel time	239 m/sec	MV annulus	cm
MV pt ½	ms	LV dP/dt	mmHg/sec	Regurgitation	trivial
Peak gradient	mmHg	Mean grad	mmHg	MV VTI	
Valve area	cm^2			Stenosis	nil

The measurements seen on the mitral valve section mostly relate to the characterisation of the diastolic function of the LV, which should be displayed in the summary of the report if you need to comment on it. The important information from this section should relate to the degree of regurgitation (trivial in this example) and the degree of stenosis. Stenosis will be quantified on the basis of valve area (cm^2) and mean gradient (mmHg), the significant ranges of which are summarised in Table 6.7 on page 160.

Tricuspid valve Doppler haemodynamics

TABLE 6.4 Doppler haemodynamics: Tricuspid valve

Vmax	1.9 m/sec	Peak gradient	15 mmHg	Est RA pres	10 mmHg
TV annulus	cm	RVSP	25 mmHg	Regurgitation	trivial
IVC	cm	% collapse		Stenosis	nil

Most people have a degree of tricuspid regurgitation. Looking at the tricuspid valve Doppler information is required to estimate the pulmonary artery systolic pressure, which essentially equates to the right ventricular systolic pressure (RVSP). A degree of regurgitation allows the calculation of the gradient across the tricuspid valve (15 mmHg in this case). The size and respiratory variation in the inferior vena cava allows a guess at the right atrial pressure (10 mmHg in this case). These two numbers are added to get the RVSP (25 mmHg).

Pulmonary vein and myocardium

TABLE 6.5 Doppler haemodynamics: Pulmonary vein and myocardium

Pulmonary vein					
S	0.7 m/sec	D	0.5 m/sec	A	0.2 m/sec
Tissue Doppler					
S'	cm/sec	A'	cm/sec	E'	10.0 cm/sec
E/E'	9				

Quantification of the blood-flow pattern through the pulmonary veins is undertaken mainly to indicate changes in the left atrial pressure. In simple terms, if the systolic (S) component is larger than the diastolic (D) component the LA pressure is likely to be normal (as in this case).

Tissue Doppler of the myocardium below the mitral annulus detects the direction and velocity of the myocardial movement. An E' velocity of >8 cm/sec generally indicates normal diastolic function.

The state of the pulmonary valve is rarely a source of excitement in an adult echocardiography report.

Summary

The information you should be able to interpret and relate to a clinical situation includes the following:

1 *The size and structure of the relative chambers and thickness of the ventricular walls.* Enlarged atria should make you look for disease in the corresponding mitral or tricuspid valve or diastolic failure of the corresponding ventricle. A dilated ventricle will usually mean failure or volume overload, and hypertrophy of the ventricular wall will usually mean pressure overload (hypertension or valve stenosis). Check for asymmetrical or septal hypertrophy of the left ventricle as this may represent hypertrophic obstructive cardiomyopathy (HOCM).

2 *The systolic function of the left ventricle.* This is generally expressed as an ejection fraction, which is the percentage of the left ventricular diastolic volume that is ejected in systole. Normally it is around 60%, and less than 50% is abnormal. Numbers less than 40% are clearly significant and deserving of comment.

Reports will often quote a fractional shortening, which is the change in the internal diameter of the base of the left ventricle from diastole to systole (normal range 28–44%). It is contingent on a single measurement and should not be seen as being as reliable as a properly calculated ejection fraction. This number will be quoted in the M-mode assessment section of the report, often associated with an ejection fraction that may be generated from cubing the same basic dimensional change. There will often be a more reliable ejection fraction quoted later in the report that is calculated by tracing the endocardial border of the left ventricle.

Also related to the left ventricle is the presence or absence of regional wall motion abnormalities. These usually relate to ischaemia or infarction as a result of coronary artery disease, and should be detailed in the report summary. The aim of a stress echo is to induce these changes to indicate myocardium that is at risk of infarction.

3 *The systolic function of the right ventricle.* The geometry for the chamber makes this difficult to accurately quantify, so you will usually see qualitative statements, such as normal or reduced.

Coupled with the state of the right ventricle is assessment of the pulmonary artery pressure, the calculation of which is discussed above. The normal value is 25 mmHg, and pulmonary hypertension should be anticipated in those patients with mitral valve disease, left ventricular failure, respiratory failure or sleep apnoea, all of which are common medical viva cases.

4 *The diastolic function or 'stiffness' of the left ventricle.* This is graded according to a range of parameters including mitral inflow patterns, pulmonary vein flow, and the movement of the myocardium below the mitral annulus.

The grading may be expressed in the report as grade I to grade IV diastolic function. Grade I relates to impaired relaxation of the ventricle without a rise in left atrial pressure. Pseudonormal (grade II) and restrictive (grade III and IV) diastolic dysfunction are of increasing severity with raised LA pressure. Such patients will operate on a higher and narrower part of the Frank-Starling curve, are more prone to hypotension with blood loss or vasodilatation, and more easily develop pulmonary oedema with fluid overload. This is clearly important information which the examiners may be keen for you to expand upon.

5 *The state of the valves, detailing their morphology and degree of regurgitation or stenosis.* You should have some understanding as to how these are quantified and their significance to anaesthesia. Valve lesions provide good medical viva cases as they have signs that you are expected to elicit and interpret, so the echo report is bound to follow. Remember that in general a stenotic lesion represents a greater danger to the anaesthetised patient (and the candidate) than a regurgitant lesion.

The severity of a valve stenosis will usually be quantified in the echo report on the basis of a pressure gradient across the valve, or as a cross-sectional area of the valve. The cross-sectional area number will always be the more reliable, as the pressure gradient is dependent on flow (the cardiac output). A failing heart will produce a lower gradient for a similar degree of stenosis.

6 *The state of the pericardium.* This will be either thickened, potentially representing constrictive pericarditis, or contain fluid, which may be at risk of cardiac tamponade. Some understanding of the signs of tamponade (chamber collapse in diastole) and its significance in anaesthesia and positive pressure ventilation is required. Such cases may be coupled with characteristic ECGs or chest X-rays.

On the following pages are a number of sample echo reports. Brief answers are given on pages 196–7.

TABLE 6.6 Grading of aortic stenosis

Degree of aortic stenosis	Peak gradient (mmHg)	Mean gradient (mmHg)	Valve area (cm²)
Normal			>2.5
Mild	25–50	12–25	1.2–1.8
Moderate	50–80	25–40	0.8–1.2
Severe	>80	40–50	0.6–0.8
Critical	>100	>50	<0.6

TABLE 6.7 Grading of mitral stenosis

Degree of mitral stenosis	Mean transvalvular pressure gradient (mmHg)	Mitral valve area (cm²)
Normal		4–6
Mild	<5	>1.5
Moderate	5–10	1.0–1.5
Severe	>10	<1.0

Case 21

This 75-year-old female patient with a history of angina presents with a fractured hip following a syncopal episode. Examination reveals a loud ejection systolic murmur. The ECG shows ST depression and evidence of left ventricular hypertrophy.

TABLE 6.8

M-mode measurements

LVIDd	4.7 cm	Left atrium	4.0 cm	LV mass	335 gm
LVIDs	3.1 cm	Aortic root	2.0 cm	LV mass (corrected)	gm
IVS	1.7 cm	LA:Ao ratio	2.0	Dia vol	104 mL
Posterior wall	1.5 cm	Right ventricle	3.3 cm	Sys vol	38 mL
FS	34%	SV	65 mL	EF	63%
Prox Asc Aorta:	cm				

Doppler haemodynamics

Aortic valve

V2 (Vmax)	5.7 m/sec	Peak gradient	132 mmHg	Aortic V2 VTI	146 cm
Mean gradient	75 mmHg	AVA max	0.34 cm^2	AVA VTI	0.4 cm^2
LVOT diameter	1.9 cm	LVOT (VTI)	18.0 cm	Regurgitation	mild
AR pt1/2	ms	AI slope	m/sec^2	Stenosis	severe

Mitral valve

E wave	1.0 m/sec	A wave	0.4 m/sec	E:A ratio	2.5
A wave duration	ms	Decel time	140 m/sec	MV annulus	cm
MV pt ½	41 ms	LV dP/dt	mmHg/sec	Regurgitation	mild
Peak gradient	mmHg	Mean grad	mmHg	MV VTI	
Area	5.4 cm^2			Stenosis	nil

Tricuspid valve

Vmax:	3.0 m/sec	Peak gradient	36 mmHg	Est RA Pres	10 mmHg
TV annulus	cm	RVSP	46 mmHg	Regurgitation	mild
IVC	cm	% collapse		Stenosis	nil

Pulmonary vein

S	0.4 m/sec	D	0.6 m/sec	A	0.4 m/sec

Tissue Doppler

S'	cm/sec	A'	cm/sec	E'	6 cm/sec
E/E'	16.6				

Summary	Heavily calcified tricuspid aortic valve. Preserved LV systolic function, no regional wall abnormalities seen. Type II diastolic dysfunction.

a Outline the principal echocardiography findings.
b Discuss your perioperative management.

Case 22

A 60-year-old man with a history of diabetes presents with shortness of breath. Examination reveals basal lung crepitations and a soft systolic murmur radiating to the apex.

TABLE 6.9

M-Mode measurements

LVIDd	7.0 cm	Left atrium	5.0 cm	LV mass	gm
LVIDs	6.0 cm	Aortic root	2.5 cm	LV mass (corrected)	gm
IVS	1.0 cm	LA:Ao ratio	2.0	Dia vol	207 mL
Posterior wall	1.1 cm	Right ventricle	cm	Sys vol	mL
FS	7%	SV	42 mL	EF	16%
Prox asc aorta:	cm				

Doppler haemodynamics

Aortic valve

V2 (Vmax)	1.2 m/sec	Peak gradient	mmHg	Aortic V2 VTI	30.0 cm
Mean gradient	mmHg	AVA max:	cm²	AVA VTI	2.6 cm²
LVOT diameter	2.5 cm	LVOT (VTI)	16.0 cm	Regurgitation	trivial
AR pt1/2	ms	AI slope	m/sec²	Stenosis	

Mitral valve

E wave	1.2 m/sec	A wave	0.4 m/sec	E:A ratio	3
A wave duration	ms	Decel time	m/sec	MV Annulus	cm
MV pt ½	ms	LV dP/dt	mmHg/sec	Regurgitation	mod
Peak gradient	mmHg	Mean grad	mmHg	MV VTI	
Area	cm²			Stenosis	nil

Tricuspid valve

Vmax:	2.5 m/sec	Peak gradient	25 mmHg	Est RA pres	15 mmHg
TV annulus	cm	RVSP	40 mmHg	Regurgitation	mild
IVC	cm	% collapse		Stenosis	nil

Pulmonary vein

S	0.3 m/sec	D	0.6 m/sec	A	0.4 m/sec

Tissue Doppler

S'	cm/sec	A'	cm/sec	E'	6 cm/sec
E/E'					

Summary	Left ventricular apical dyskinesis, antero-lateral akinesis, EF by Simpsons method 14%
	Central mitral regurgitation, normal leaflets.

a Describe the echocardiographic abnormalities.
b What is the most likely mechanism of this patient's heart failure?

Case 23

A 25-year-old primigravid woman presents at 26 weeks pregnant with increasing shortness of breath. ECG reveals atrial fibrillation.

TABLE 6.10

M-mode measurements				
LVIDd	3.5 cm	Left atrium	5.0 cm	LV mass	gm
LVIDs	2.5 cm	Aortic root	2.5 cm	LV mass (corrected)	gm
IVS	1.0 cm	LA:Ao ratio	2.0	Dia vol	mL
Posterior wall	0.9 cm	Right ventricle	cm	Sys vol	mL
FS	28%	SV	mL	EF	
Prox asc aorta:	cm				

Doppler haemodynamics				

Aortic valve				
V2 (Vmax)	1.2 m/sec	Peak gradient	6 mmHg	Aortic V2 VTI	cm
Mean gradient	4 mmHg	AVA max:	cm^2	AVA VTI	cm^2
LVOT diameter	2.0 cm	LVOT (VTI)	cm	Regurgitation	trivial
AR pt1/2	ms	AI slope	m/sec^2	Stenosis	nil

Mitral valve				
E wave	2.0 m/sec	A wave	m/sec	E:A ratio	
A wave duration	ms	Decel time	820 m/sec	MV Annulus	cm
MV pt ½	240 ms	LV dP/dt	mmHg/sec	Regurgitation	mild
Peak gradient	16 mmHg	Mean grad	11 mmHg	MV VTI	
Area	0.9 cm^2			Stenosis	severe

Tricuspid valve				
Vmax:	2.9 m/sec	Peak gradient	35 mmHg	Est RA pres	15 mmHg
TV annulus	cm	RVSP	50 mmHg	Regurgitation	mod
IVC	cm	% collapse		Stenosis	nil

Pulmonary vein				
S	m/sec	D	m/sec	A	m/sec

Tissue Doppler				
S'	cm/sec	A'	cm/sec	E'	cm/sec
E/E'					

Summary	Thickened mitral leaflets, diastolic doming. Dilated LA, LV. Atrial fibrillation.

a What are the major echocardiographic findings?
b What is the likely cause?
c How would you manage her delivery?

Case 24

A 40-year-old man was noted to have a heart murmur as a child, and has been having regular echocardiography. Physical examination reveals an early diastolic murmur at the left sternal edge.

TABLE 6.11

M-mode measurements					
LVIDd	5.5 cm	Left atrium	4.0 cm	LV mass	gm
LVIDs	3.5 cm	Aortic root	4.0 cm	LV mass (corrected)	gm
IVS	1.2 cm	LA:Ao ratio	1.0	Dia vol	mL
Posterior wall	1.2 cm	Right ventricle	cm	Sys vol	mL
FS	36%	SV	56 mL	EF:	67%
Prox asc aorta:	5.0 cm				

Doppler haemodynamics					
Aortic valve					
V2 (Vmax)	1.9 m/sec	Peak gradient	mmHg	Aortic V2 VTI	29.0 cm
Mean gradient	mmHg	AVA max:	cm²	AVA VTI	cm²
LVOT diameter	2.5 cm	LVOT (VTI)	20.0 cm	Regurgitation	severe
AR pt1/2	200 ms	AI slope	m/sec²	Stenosis	nil

Mitral valve					
E wave	0.8 m/sec	A wave	0.5 m/sec	E:A ratio	1.6
A wave duration	ms	Decel time	220 m/sec	MV annulus	cm
MV pt ½	ms	LV dP/dt	mmHg/sec	Regurgitation	mild
Peak gradient	mmHg	Mean grad	mmHg	MV VTI	
Area	cm²			Stenosis	nil

Tricuspid valve					
Vmax:	2.1 m/sec	Peak gradient	18 mmHg	Est RA pres	5 mmHg
TV annulus	cm	RVSP	23 mmHg	Regurgitation	trivial
IVC	cm	% collapse		Stenosis	nil

Pulmonary vein					
S	0.7 m/sec	D		0.5 m/sec	A	0.2 m/sec

Tissue Doppler					
S'	cm/sec	A'	cm/sec	E'	10.0 cm/sec
E/E'	9				
Summary	Bicuspid aortic valve				

a What are the echocardiographic abnormalities?
b What procedure does this patient likely require?

Case 25

A previously well 30-year-old female presents with a slow onset of shortness of breath and vague chest pain. Physical examination reveals a parasternal heave and a loud second heart sound.

TABLE 6.12

M-mode measurements

LVIDd	3.5 cm	Left atrium	3.3 cm	LV mass	gm
LVIDs	2.5 cm	Aortic root	2.0 cm	LV mass (corrected)	gm
IVS	1.3 cm	LA:Ao ratio	1.65	Dia vol	mL
Posterior wall	1.0 cm	Right ventricle	4.5 cm	Sys vol	mL
FS	29%	SV	ml	EF:	62%
Prox asc aorta:	cm				

Doppler haemodynamics

Aortic valve

V2 (Vmax)	1.3 m/sec	Peak gradient	mmHg	Aortic V2 VTI	cm
Mean gradient	mmHg	AVA max:	cm²	AVA VTI	cm²
LVOT diameter	2.0 cm	LVOT (VTI)	cm	Regurgitation	nil
AR pt1/2	ms	AI slope	m/sec²	Stenosis	nil

Mitral valve

E wave	0.8 m/sec	A wave	0.5 m/sec	E:A ratio	1.6
A wave duration	ms	Decel time	m/sec	MV annulus	cm
MV pt ½	ms	LV dP/dt	mmHg/sec	Regurgitation	nil
Peak gradient	mmHg	Mean grad	mmHg	MV VTI	
Area	cm²			Stenosis	nil

Tricuspid valve

Vmax:	3.5 m/sec	Peak gradient	49 mmHg	Est RA pres	15 mmHg
TV annulus	cm	RVSP	64 mmHg	Regurgitation	mod
IVC	cm	% collapse		Stenosis	nil

Pulmonary vein

S	0.5 m/sec	D	0.5 m/sec	A	0.2 m/sec

Tissue Doppler

S'	cm/sec	A'	cm/sec	E'	10.0 cm/sec
E/E'					

Summary	Hypertrophic right ventricular wall. Systolic flattening of interventricular septum, interatrial septum appears intact. Pulmonary valve appears normal.

a What is the main echocardiographic abnormality?
b What are the possible underlying causes?

Case 26

A 20-year-old man was told he had a heart murmur as a child but was lost to follow-up. On presentation to a pre-admission clinic he is noted to have a mid-systolic murmur and an obviously split second heart sound.

TABLE 6.13

M-mode measurements					
LVIDd	4.6 cm	Left atrium	3.7 cm	LV mass	gm
LVIDs	2.8 cm	Aortic root	2.8 cm	LV mass (corrected)	gm
IVS	1.0 cm	LA:Ao ratio	1.32	Dia vol	89 mL
Posterior wall	1.0 cm	Right ventricle	cm	Sys vol	28 mL
FS	39%	SV	mL	EF:	69%
Prox asc aorta:	cm				

Doppler haemodynamics					
Aortic valve					
V2 (Vmax)	1.2 m/sec	Peak gradient	mmHg	Aortic V2 VTI	cm
Mean gradient	mmHg	AVA max:	cm²	AVA VTI	cm²
LVOT diameter	cm	LVOT (VTI)	cm	Regurgitation	trivial
AR pt1/2	ms	AI slope	m/sec²	Stenosis	
Mitral valve					
E wave	0.8 m/sec	A wave	0.4 m/sec	E:A ratio	2
A wave duration	ms	Decel time	m/sec	MV annulus	cm
MV pt ½	ms	LV dP/dt	mmHg/sec	Regurgitation	trivial
Peak gradient	mmHg	Mean grad	mmHg	MV VTI	
Area	cm²			Stenosis	nil
Tricuspid valve					
Vmax:	m/sec	Peak gradient	30 mmHg	Est RA pres	5 mmHg
TV annulus	cm	RVSP	35 mmHg	Regurgitation	mild
IVC	cm	% collapse		Stenosis	nil
Pulmonary vein					
S	0.6 m/sec	D	0.3 m/sec	A	0.2 m/sec
Tissue Doppler					
S'	cm/sec	A'	cm/sec	E'	cm/sec
E/E'	9				
Summary	2 cm ASD, left to right shunt, mildly dilated RA, RV Qp:Qs 4.0				

a Discuss the meaning of Qp:Qs ratio.
b At what stage should the ASD be repaired?

7. Arterial blood gas analysis

Overview

When presented with arterial blood gas results in the examination always consider these in conjunction with the clinical scenario presented. Use all of the information available to arrive at an acid-base diagnosis, and consider how this may have arisen in the given situation. Candidates should have a comprehensive list of differential diagnoses for major metabolic and respiratory abnormalities. Remember that arterial blood gases also provide useful insight into the oxygenation of the patient!

For all biochemical data, reference ranges should always be provided in the exam. Evaluation of the pH, pCO_2 and bicarbonate will usually give you enough information to determine the likely primary process. Always assess the magnitude of any compensatory response and its adequacy. Remember that more than one primary process may be present, so be alert to the possibility of a mixed picture. However, within the limitations of the examination process it is unlikely that an extremely complicated combination of acid-base abnormalities will be presented in the one example. You may be expected to provide a more considered analysis if the data are presented as part of the clinical scenario preceding an anaesthesia viva (when the time before the bell signalling the start of the viva can be spent calculating anion gaps and expected values for compensatory responses).

Once an acid-base diagnosis is established, formulate a differential diagnosis and consider what other tests might be needed to make a definitive clinical diagnosis, and how you would approach the management of the patient.

An outline of a possible approach to acid-base disorders is provided below, with several examples. For those seeking a more comprehensive analysis of the topic, Dr Kerry Brandis' treatise on acid-base physiology (available online at www.anaesthesiamcq.com/AcidBaseBook) has attracted international renown, and is an essential reference.

Ancillary calculations

When a metabolic acidosis is diagnosed, it is useful to calculate the anion gap (AG):

$$AG = ([Na^+] + [K^+]) - ([Cl^-] + [HCO3^-]) \text{ mmol/L (normal: } 8 - 16 \text{ mmol/L)}$$

Causes of a normal anion gap metabolic acidosis include gastrointestinal loss of bicarbonate, renal tubular acidosis and hyperchloraemia.

Causes of an increased anion gap metabolic acidosis include lactic acidosis, ketoacidosis, renal failure and exogenous toxic alcohols.

The measurement of oxygen on blood gas determinations should not be ignored; inference can be made as to the presence and effectiveness of supplemental oxygen administration.

The Alveolar–arterial gradient for oxygen ($P_AO_2 - PaO_2$) can also be calculated and may be useful in determining the aetiology of hypoxaemia (PaO_2 is measured):

$$P_AO_2 = P_{inspired} O_2 - PCO_2 / R \text{ (alveolar gas equation), where}$$

$$P_{inspired} O_2 = F_{inspired} O_2 \times (P_{ATM} - \text{Saturated Vapour Pressure}_{H_2O}).$$

The normal A–a gradient is less than 10 mmHg, but increases with age and as F_IO_2 increases. For practical purposes, rapid calculations making use of A–a gradients are unlikely in the clinical components of the exam.

One suggested system for ABG analysis is given in Box 6.4.

BOX 6.4 System for ABG analysis

1. Demographic and technical aspects
   - Patient ID, date, time of collection
   - Patient temperature
   - F_IO_2

2. Consider the pH
   - If low, an acidosis must be present.
   - If high, an alkalosis must be present.
   - If normal, either no disorder or mixed disorder.
   - Note that mixed disorder may be present in all three cases.

3. Is the primary disorder respiratory or metabolic? Consider the $[HCO_3^-]$ and pCO_2
   - If both are high, suggests respiratory acidosis or metabolic alkalosis.
   - If both are low, suggests respiratory alkalosis or metabolic acidosis.
   - If they move in opposite directions, a mixed disorder must be present.

4. Is the compensatory response appropriate? If varies from expected result, mixed disorder likely
   - For acute respiratory acidosis: expected $[HCO_3^-] = 24 + (pCO_2 - 40)/10$ mmol/L
   - For chronic respiratory acidosis: expected $[HCO_3^-] = 24 + 4 \times (pCO_2 - 40)/10$ mmol/L
   - For acute respiratory alkalosis: expected $[HCO_3^-] = 24 - 2 \times (40 - pCO_2)/10$ mmol/L
   - For chronic respiratory alkalosis: expected $[HCO_3^-] = 24 - 5 \times (40 - pCO_2)/10$ mmol/L
   - For metabolic acidosis: expected $pCO_2 = 1.5 \times [HCO_3^-] + 8$ mmHg
   - For metabolic alkalosis: expected $pCO_2 = 0.7 \times [HCO_3^-] + 20$ mmHg

5. Further evaluation
   - Is diagnosis consistent with history and examination?
   - Is any other information available?
   - What further tests are needed to confirm the diagnosis?

The following pages contain examples that are representative of the types of questions you might expect in the vivas. Answers can be found on page 197.

Case 27

A 22-year-old man is brought into the emergency department complaining of nausea and abdominal pain. He looks extremely unwell and appears confused. The following blood tests are obtained:

TABLE 6.14

Arterial blood gas			Serum biochemistry		
Sample	Ref range		Sample	Ref range	
pH	7.13	(7.35–7.45)	Sodium	136 mmol/L	(137–145)
pO$_2$	85 mmHg	(80–95)	Potassium	6.4 mmol/L	(3.5–5.0)
pCO$_2$	16 mmHg	(35–45)	Chloride	92 mmol/L	(98–106)
HCO$_3$$^-$	5.2 mmol/L	(22–26)	Glucose	39 mmol/L	(3.5–6.0)

a What is the most likely clinical diagnosis?
b What acid-base disorder is present?
c What other tests would you perform on this patient?
d Outline your management strategies for this patient.

Case 28

You receive handover of general anaesthesia from a colleague who is fatigued. The patient is a 65-year-old man undergoing radical retropubic prostatectomy. He is otherwise well. An arterial blood sample analysis from the patient midway through the procedure is as follows:

TABLE 6.15 Arterial blood gas

	Sample	Ref range
pH	7.58	(7.35–7.45)
pO$_2$	165 mmHg	(80–95)
pCO$_2$	22 mmHg	(35–45)
HCO$_3$$^-$	20.4 mmol/L	(22–26)

a What acid-base disorder is present?
b How would you investigate and remedy this problem?

Case 29

A 78-year-old patient is transferred from a peripheral regional hospital to your tertiary centre for emergency surgery to relieve a small bowel obstruction. The patient has been vomiting for several days, but on arrival is haemodynamically stable and appears comfortable. As part of a preoperative work-up the following blood gas analysis is performed:

TABLE 6.16 Arterial blood gas		
	Sample	Ref range
pH	7.48	(7.35–7.45)
pO_2	75 mmHg	(80–95)
pCO_2	61.1 mmHg	(35–45)
HCO_3^-	42.6 mmol/L	(22–26)

a Comment on the acid-base status of the patient.
b Are these results consistent with your expectations?
c Formulate a plan for the fluid management in the perioperative period for this patient.

Case 30

A 69-year-old with long-standing emphysema presents with lethargy and anorexia. Arterial blood gas analysis is performed as follows:

TABLE 6.17 Arterial blood gas		
	Sample	Ref range
pH	7.22	(7.35–7.45)
pO_2	49 mmHg	(80–95)
pCO_2	58.3 mmHg	(35–45)
HCO_3^-	24.2 mmol/L	(22–26)

a What is your acid-base diagnosis in this patient?
b What other biochemical tests would you order?

8. Coagulation studies

Overview

Coagulation studies may appear in anaesthesia vivas and medical vivas in several situations. Firstly, they may be part of the preoperative investigation of a patient with a history of pathological bleeding (inherited or acquired). The candidate would be expected to interpret the results in significant conditions such as liver disease, von Willebrand's disease or haemophilia. Secondly, it is important for candidates to have a good grasp of the perioperative management of patients with impaired coagulation. Typical situations, such as the reversal of the anticoagulation of a patient on warfarin therapy, central neuraxial block, and acquired conditions such as severe pre-eclampsia, are core material. Finally, the management of blood component therapy in the situation of massive haemorrhage clearly requires an understanding of the coagulation changes expected and an idea of how to go about correcting them.

The classical extrinsic and intrinsic pathway mechanism that was traditionally taught in the basic sciences probably does not occur in vivo. This cascade concept has been replaced by the cell-based model of haemostasis, which describes the process as occurring on cell surfaces as three overlapping steps. Firstly, initiation relies on the exposure of cells bearing tissue factor, which in several steps release a 'priming' dose of thrombin. The amplification phase involves platelets and cofactors being activated to prepare for large-scale thrombin generation. Finally, in the amplification phase large amounts of thrombin are generated on the platelet surface.

The coagulation profile is a relatively poor routine preoperative screening test, with low sensitivity and specificity for detecting mild derangements in coagulation. It is also important to remember that it only tells you about platelet number, not function. This clearly has implications for the patient on anti-platelet agents such as aspirin or clopidogrel, where the coagulation profile would be expected to be normal.

The standard coagulation studies are expected to include:

- prothrombin time (PT)
- activated partial thromboplastin time (aPTT)
- fibrinogen
- platelet count.

Other basic tests that have a place in the preoperative management of coagulopathy are platelet function analysis, thromboelastography and activated coagulation time (ACT).

Remember that in the exam the laboratory result should be accompanied by the reference range.

Prothrombin time (PT)

The prothrombin time is measured by re-calcifying platelet-poor plasma at 37°C in the presence of a reagent with tissue factor activity and measuring the time to clot formation. The normal time is usually 11 to 15 seconds, but this is dependent on the nature of the reagent used. For this reason, when following the therapeutic effect of oral anticoagulant medication, it is best expressed as the ratio to a control, the international normalised ratio (INR).

The traditional teaching is that the prothrombin time tests the extrinsic and common pathways of the coagulation system, i.e. factors I, II, V, VII and X. The main causes of a prolonged prothrombin time are warfarin therapy, liver disease, malabsorption of vitamin K, and disseminated intravascular coagulation.

Activated partial thromboplastin time (aPTT)

The aPTT is also measured by the re-calcification of platelet-poor plasma at 37°C, but in the presence of an activator and platelet substitute, measuring the time for the sample of plasma to clot. The reference range is usually 25 to 30 seconds. It is traditionally considered to be a measure of the function of the intrinsic and common pathway, as well as the means of monitoring the therapeutic effect of unfractionated heparin therapy.

An isolated prolongation of the aPTT suggests a deficiency of factor VIII (including von Willebrand's disease), factor IX, factor XI or factor XII. A prolongation of both the PT and the aPTT suggests a deficiency of factor I (fibrinogen), factor II, factor V or factor X. It will also be prolonged with heparin therapy, lupus inhibitor, liver disease and disseminated intravascular coagulation.

Platelet count

The platelet count is automatically measured as part of a standard full blood count examination. It may be manually checked by microscopy, in which the presence of clumping of platelets indicates that the low platelet count is probably artifactual. The normal range is 150–400 $\times 10^9$/litre.

Occasionally the platelet count will be elevated in the perioperative patient. The usual reason for this is a reactive rise in response to sepsis or trauma. Occasionally it will be due to essential thrombocythaemia, which is a myeloproliferative disease in which neoplastic haemopoietic stem cell proliferation leads to an increase in platelet production.

Thrombocytopaenia is a platelet count below 150×10^9/litre; however, it is of little clinical impact until the count falls below 100×10^9/litre. A low platelet count is either the result of a failure of marrow production, usually as part of a pancytopaenia (often drug effects or malignancy), or as a result of increased peripheral destruction. Peripheral destruction can be immune mediated, as in autoimmune diseases, or relate to the development of drug-dependent antiplatelet antibodies, of which heparin is the example of most anaesthesia concern. Some critically ill perioperative patients will develop a consumptive thrombocytopaenia as part of a disseminated intravascular coagulation. A similar process of consumption combined with dilution is seen in massive transfusion. The analysis of platelet function is discussed below.

Fibrinogen

Fibrinogen (factor I) conversion to fibrin is the final step in the coagulation pathway. The normal range for fibrinogen is 1.5 to 4 grams/litre.

The fibrinogen level is often elevated as part of an acute phase response, which is common following surgery. Low levels indicate decreased production (liver disease or rare inherited deficiency) or increased consumption (disseminated intravascular coagulation or fibrinolysis).

The increased popularity of the massive transfusion protocol to guide the blood component replacement in the face of major blood loss frequently mandates the use of cryoprecipitate to restore fibrinogen levels. The increased role of fibrinogen replacement in the bleeding patient means that it is an obvious topic of discussion in a viva.

Prothrombotic disorders should be suspected in patients with episodes of recurrent thromboembolism, especially if it occurs in young adults. There may be a family history of protein C, protein S and antithrombin III deficiency.

Platelet function

Although the platelet count is useful in situations of quantitative platelet defects, many of the disease processes and medication effects on the platelet result in a normal count with a functional defect. These are traditionally difficult to quantify and there appears to be no clear consensus regarding the best method.

The in vivo bleeding time was the first method available for the testing of platelet function. It was standardised as the Modified Ivy bleeding time, where a sphygmomanometer is inflated on the upper arm to a pressure of 40 mmHg, and a standardised superficial incision in the skin is made on the volar aspect of the forearm with a commercial disposable device. The time to the cessation of bleeding is recorded, with a normal being less than 9 minutes. The test is very operator dependent, is neither sensitive nor specific for the risk of operative bleeding and is poorly reproducible. It is also impractical for serial measurements to be obtained during a procedure. Increasingly, the test is not being offered by laboratories, but it is still frequently mentioned in anaesthesia texts.

A range of other platelet function tests are variably available, including Platelet Function Analyser (PFA-100), platelet aggregometry and flow cytometry. The

PFA-100 system seems to be the most popular means of screening for platelet dysfunction, and is relatively simple to perform from a laboratory point of view. It produces a value called the closure time, which represents the time to haemostatic plug formation within the centre of a membrane coated with collagen and either ADP or epinephrine. A normal col/epi closure time (<183 sec) excludes a significant platelet function defect. If the col/epi closure time is prolonged and the col/ADP closure time is normal (<122 sec), then the most likely cause of the platelet function is aspirin ingestion. The prolongation of both may indicate anaemia, thrombocytopenia or a platelet defect other than aspirin.

It is suggested that candidates be aware of the basic method of platelet analysis available at their hospital. Further testing would usually be undertaken with the advice of a haematologist.

Thromboelastography (TEG)

The thromboelastograph is a viscoelastic measure of coagulation that was developed over 60 years ago. It is regaining importance due to the development of more automated machines that allow easier bedside evaluation of coagulation. The classic method involves the placement of 0.36 mL of whole blood in a cuvette. This cuvette oscillates on its axis every 10 seconds through an arc of approximately 5°. As the clot develops, the rotation is transferred to a pin immersed in the sample and this movement is electronically recorded on a graph. This has been modified with the rotational thromboelastograph (ROTEM), where the sensor shaft rotates instead of the sample. This method is said to be more reliable and reproducible.

The process produces a cigar-shaped graph, and records the dynamics of the clot formation. It is able to differentiate the various causes of failed haemostasis, including platelet defects, coagulation factor deficiency and fibrinolysis. It is becoming frequently used in liver transplantation and cardiac surgery and as automated TEG systems increase in popularity it would be reasonable for FANZCA candidates to be able to discuss the basics of the test.

The parameters that are calculated from the TEG include the following and are represented in Figure 6.55a and b (below and opposite). The normal values are included as a guide, but they are variable between institutions and on the presence of the activator that is used in the sample.

- R time – the time from test initiation to the first formation of fibrin. (RR 4–8 min)
- K – the measure of time from the beginning of clot formation until the amplitude of the thromboelastogram reaches 20 mm, representing the dynamics of the clot formation. (RR 1–4 min)

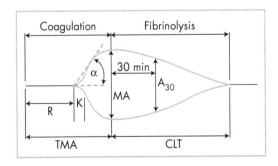

(a) The major features of a thromboelastograph trace

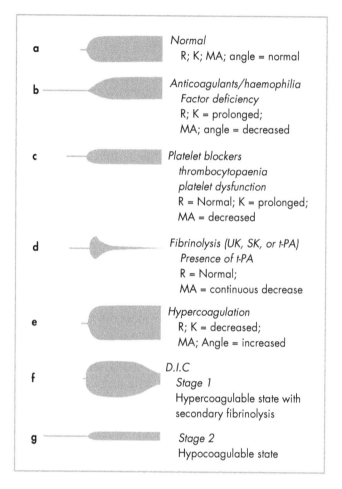

a   *Normal*
R; K; MA; angle = normal

b   *Anticoagulants/haemophilia*
Factor deficiency
R; K = prolonged;
MA; angle = decreased

c   *Platelet blockers*
thrombocytopaenia
platelet dysfunction
R = Normal; K = prolonged;
MA = decreased

d   *Fibrinolysis (UK, SK, or t-PA)*
Presence of t-PA
R = Normal;
MA = continuous decrease

e   *Hypercoagulation*
R; K = decreased;
MA; Angle = increased

f   *D.I.C*
Stage 1
Hypercoagulable state with
secondary fibrinolysis

g   *Stage 2*
Hypocoagulable state

(b) A sample of representative traces for commonly seen clotting disorders

- Alpha angle – tangential to the developing body of the graph, indicating the kinetics of fibrin build-up and cross linking. (RR 47–74°)
- MA or maximum amplitude – represents the maximum strength of the clot. (RR 55–73 mm)
- A_{30} – the amplitude at 30 minutes, indicating the stability of the clot (sometimes measured at 60 minutes). A high rate of decline following the MA is indicative of fibrinolysis.

Activated coagulation (clotting) time (ACT)

The ACT is typically used in anaesthesia practice as a means of monitoring the degree of heparinisation for cardiopulmonary bypass. A whole blood sample is 'activated' with either kaolin or celite (diatomaceous earth). Its advantage is its ease of use at the bedside and the relative linearity of the result with large doses of heparin. The normal or baseline result is typically around 120 seconds, and this is relatively insensitive to platelet dysfunction. Most anaesthetists would insist on a value of at least 400 seconds before going on bypass.

The following cases contain examples of typical coagulation studies. The answers are on page 198.

Case 31

This coagulation profile is a preoperative sample from a menorrhagic 35-year-old woman booked for a total abdominal hysterectomy.

TABLE 6.18

	Sample	Ref range
PT	12 sec	(11–15 sec)
INR	1.0	
aPTT	45 sec	(25–35 sec)
Fibrinogen	3.0 g/L	(1.5–4 g/L)
Platelets	240 x 10⁹/L	(150 – 400 × 10⁹/L)

a What is the likely diagnosis and how could it be investigated further?
b How would you manage the problem perioperatively?

Case 32

A 24-year-old previously well primiparous woman suddenly collapses in the third stage of labour. The following coagulation profile was obtained:

TABLE 6.19

	Sample	Ref range
PT	30 sec	(11–15 sec)
INR	2.7	
aPTT	90 sec	(25–35 sec)
Fibrinogen	0.5 g/L	(1.5–4 g/L)
Platelets	40 × 10⁹/L	(150 – 400 × 10⁹/L)

a What is the diagnosis?
b What is the nature of the coagulopathy?

Case 33

A previously well patient develops biliary colic, and then becomes jaundiced. He is referred for ERCP and this coagulation profile is obtained.

TABLE 6.20

	Sample	Ref range
PT	24 sec	(11–15 sec)
INR	2.0	
aPTT	55 sec	(25–35 sec)
Fibrinogen	3.5 g/L	(1.5–4 g/L)
Platelets	200 × 10⁹/L	(150 – 400 × 10⁹/L)

a What is the mechanism of the coagulation disturbance?
b How would you manage the coagulopathy?

Case 34

A young woman is scheduled for a splenectomy for refractory thrombocytopenia.

TABLE 6.21

	Sample	Ref range
PT	13 sec	(11–15 sec)
INR	1.2	
aPTT	34 sec	(25–35 sec)
Fibrinogen	3.1 g/L	(1.5–4 g/L)
Platelets	12×10^9/L	$(150 - 400 \times 10^9$/L)

a What is the disease and mechanism of the thrombocytopenia?
b Outline the perioperative management of this patient.

Case 35

A 50-year-old man with a previous history of alcohol abuse presents with haematemesis.

TABLE 6.22

	Sample	Ref range
PT	25 sec	(11–15 sec)
INR	2.2	
aPTT	51 sec	(25–35 sec)
Fibrinogen	0.9 g/L	(1.5–4 g/L)
Platelets	90×10^9/L	$(150 - 400 \times 10^9$/L)

a What is the mechanism of his coagulopathy?
b How would you manage his coagulopathy?

9. Full blood count examination

The full blood count is such a common investigation in the perioperative patient that rapid and accurate interpretation of the result is expected in the final anaesthesia exam. As with any investigation the interpretation must first and foremost be in light of the clinical scenario presented, looking for the obvious expected abnormalities. Vocalising these may well prompt the examiner to move on to other material. If not, the interpretation should then follow a systematic approach to identify further abnormalities.

The full blood count requires an EDTA (i.e. unclotted) blood sample that is automatically analysed. This automatically records (among other indices) the haemoglobin concentration, the red cell count, the white cell count, the platelet count, the mean corpuscular volume and the leukocyte differential count. The sample may also be manually examined if indicated on the basis of the automated result.

Haemoglobin

The haemoglobin concentration (normal range for men 13.5–18 g/dl; for women 11.5–16 g/dl) has obvious considerable pre- and intra-operative significance for the anaesthetist.

Preoperative anaemia requires a decision on the part of the anaesthetist as to whether to defer surgery. This represents a judgement call depending on the severity of the anaemia, the degree of surgical urgency and the prospect of timely correction of the anaemia. It is the weighing of such issues to reach a decision in the best interests of the patient that the examiners will expect from the candidate.

The cause of the anaemia is clearly important in developing a plan for its correction. This requires consideration of the clinical situation and can be narrowed somewhat by consideration of the mean corpuscular volume (MCV). The MCV represents the size of the red blood cell (normal range 80–100 fl) and largely reflects the abnormalities limiting the production of the red cell in the bone marrow. Anaemia with a low MCV occurs with iron deficiency anaemia, thalassaemia and sideroblastic anaemia. Anaemia with a high MCV occurs with folate deficiency, vitamin B_{12} deficiency, alcoholism, chronic liver disease, hypothyroidism, reticulocytosis and myelodysplasia. Anaemia with a normal MCV occurs with the anaemia of chronic disease, renal failure, pregnancy, haemolysis and marrow failure. It may also represent two underlying mechanisms with opposite effects on the size of the erythrocyte.

Perioperative anaemia also brings up the issue of transfusion triggers. Once again, this represents a judgement call on the part of the anaesthetist. The issues to be weighed in this situation are the volume status of the patient, the cardio-respiratory reserve, the probability of further (perhaps rapid) blood loss, the preoperative haemoglobin level and the current haemoglobin level. In general, haemoglobin concentrations below 7 g/dl will usually require transfusion, and levels greater than 10 g/dl will rarely indicate the need for transfusion. It is fair to say that the risks associated with blood products such as transfusion-related acute lung injury have been underestimated in the past.

Preoperative elevation of the haemoglobin concentration always deserves comment, as there is significance to the anaesthetist regardless of the cause.

'Primary' elevation is due to polycythaemia rubra vera, a myeloproliferative disease; 50% of such patients will also have an accompanying thrombocytosis. The elevation on the haemoglobin represents an increased risk for thromboembolic events in the perioperative period, and these patients should undergo venesection prior to surgery.

Secondary polycythaemia is due to the increased production of erythropoietin, which may result from renal conditions such as erythropoietin-secreting tumours or renal artery stenosis. Erythropoietin production is also increased in response to chronic hypoxaemia, the causes of which should gain the attention of the anaesthetist.

'Relative' increases in the concentration of haemoglobin relate to the loss of plasma volume (conditions such as dehydration, vomiting, fluid leakage in burns and enteropathies). Once again, these are all conditions that relate directly to the safe management of the patient during the perioperative period, and signify the need for fluid resuscitation.

White cell count

Changes in the white cell count can be caused by a myriad of factors, the listing of which is beyond the scope of this book. The following aims to give a rapid scheme for considering the major abnormalities in the exam situation.

An elevated white cell count (reference range $4.0 - 11.0 \times 10^9$/L) usually signifies an inflammatory response or the presence of infection. Elevation of the white cell count may also be the result of medication; glucocorticoid administration being the most frequent in the perioperative patient. If the white cell count is elevated always check the differential to establish which white cell line is responsible for the change. This will usually be the neutrophils in the case of bacterial infection, inflammatory response or tissue infarction.

The lymphocytes will usually be raised in response to viral infection. A monocytosis usually accompanies acute or chronic bacterial infection (including tuberculosis). An eosinophilia usually represents a chronic allergic response or a drug reaction, or a chronic parasitic infection.

It must also be remembered that elevation of a white cell line can be the result of a leukaemia or lymphoma, but these conditions do not generally rank highly in anaesthesia examinations.

The terms neutropaenia, granulocytopaenia and leukopaenia tend to be used somewhat interchangeably, but they are different and you should attempt to use the correct terminology in the exam situation. Leukopaenia refers to a reduced level of white cells in total, neutropenia refers to a decrease in the level of the neutrophils (generally defined as less than 1.5×10^9/L). Granulocytopenia refers to a reduced number of circulating cells from the granulocyte series, which includes neutrophils, eosinophils and basophils. This usually reflects the change in the number of neutrophils as these make up the bulk of the granulocytes on the normal blood film.

It is important to be able to quote a short differential diagnosis for the patient who has neutropaenia, and to be able to discuss the basic implications for anaesthesia. In hospital practice the most common cause of neutropaenia is iatrogenic, resulting from the use of cytotoxic or immunosuppressive drugs. Other causes include bone marrow failure as a result of idiosyncratic drug reactions, nutritional deficiency or infection. There may also be peripheral destruction as a result of autoimmune processes, or peripheral pooling in the case of sepsis.

As is the case with any investigation, particularly in the exam situation, the investigation result needs to be related back to the clinical scenario and interpreted on that basis.

When considering the anaesthesia implications of the neutropaenia, you need to consider the increased risk of perioperative infection, the implications for the other myeloid cell lines such as red cells and platelets, and the implications of the underlying disease process that resulted in the neutropaenia. For instance, a patient who has developed neutropaenia as a result of their chemotherapy for malignancy would need to be considered in the light of the other toxic effects of the drug, as well as the mass effects of the malignancy, the metabolic effects and the implications of possible metastatic tumour.

As a general principle, the neutropaenic patient should not be considered a surgical candidate except in an emergency.

Platelets

The implications of abnormal platelet counts were discussed in section 8, Coagulation studies.

10. Urea and electrolytes

Overview

The ordering of biochemistry on preoperative patients appears to be an unthinking and ubiquitous process that seems to occur whenever blood is drawn for some purpose. That said, there are a number of perioperative electrolyte derangements that the anaesthetist must recognise and handle with confidence. A systematic approach to the blood biochemical profile is therefore required in day-to-day work, as well as for examination purposes.

The normal blood biochemical analysis generally involves the spectrophotometry of lithium heparin blood.

In the exam situation the results should all come with reference ranges.

Sodium (Na⁺)

Sodium is the principal cation of the extracellular fluid, and is responsible for almost 90% of its osmotic activity. The normal range is 135–145 mmol/L.

Hyponatraemia is the result of sodium loss or water retention in excess of sodium, or as a combination of these two processes. The most common cause of hyponatraemia is an excess of total body water. Important causes include secretion of inappropriate antidiuretic hormone (SIADH) and TURP syndrome, where there is excess absorption of the glycine-containing irrigation solution. The important perioperative causes of sodium loss include gastrointestinal (nausea/vomiting/diarrhoea/high output fistulas), burns, diuretic use and cerebral salt wasting. All of these conditions have significant implications for the surgical patient and candidates are expected to discuss these issues in some depth.

Hyponatraemia may also appear in circumstances where the volume of the plasma is increased by hyperlipidaemia or hyperproteinaemia, and the analysis of the sample will give a lower result for all of the other measured compounds. A large quantity of osmotically active solutes that do not enter the intracellular fluid (e.g. glucose and mannitol) can lead to movement of water from the intracellular fluid to the extracellular fluid, with resultant dilution of sodium.

Hypernatraemia can be caused by the loss of water in excess of sodium or excess sodium intake or retention, or a combination of the two processes. In anaesthesia practice the dehydrated patient is a standard surgical offering where the degree of volume depletion needs to be assessed. Neurogenic diabetes insipidus is an important condition seen as a result of head injury or pituitary surgery, where decreased ADH secretion leads to renal loss of free water. The aggressive use of hypertonic saline in the setting of head injury by some intensivists is a cause of relative sodium excess.

Potassium (K⁺)

Potassium is the principal intracellular cation, and as such the serum values (RR 3.5–4.5 mmol/L) are not representative of the total body stores. As the cell membrane is significantly more permeable to the potassium ion than the sodium ion, potassium is largely responsible for the level of the resting membrane potential and hence the function of skeletal muscle, myocardium and nerves.

Because of the high intracellular concentration, haemolysis of the blood specimen will cause an artefactually high potassium concentration.

In the acute situation the relative distribution of potassium between the intracellular and extracellular fluid compartments is the major cause of changes in serum levels and is of the most importance to the anaesthetist.

Situations which promote a shift of potassium out of the cell (i.e. hyperkalaemia) include:

- acidosis
- alpha adrenergic agonists
- suxamethonium
- cell damage (rhabdomyolysis, tumour lysis, burns).

Situations which promote the shift of potassium into the cell (hypokalaemia) include:

- alkalosis
- beta 2 adrenergic agonists
- methylxanthines
- insulin.

A reduction in the total body stores of potassium will be caused by inadequate intake or increased losses. The losses will be either:

- gastrointestinal
  - vomiting, nasogastric aspiration
  - diarrhoea or enteric fistula losses

  or
- renal
  - mineralocorticoid or glucocorticoid excess
  - diuretics
  - renal tubular acidosis
  - metabolic alkalosis.

The mechanisms for the conservation of potassium by the kidney are far less efficient than those for the conservation of sodium.

An increase in the total body stores of potassium is due to either excessive intake or decreased elimination by the kidney. Causes include:

- renal failure
- potassium sparing diuretics (amiloride, spironolactone)
- ACE inhibitors
- NSAIDs
- Addison's disease, steroid withdrawal.

The clinical manifestations of severe hypokalaemia include muscle weakness, tetany, ileus, dysrhythmias and decreased cardiac contractility. The classic ECG changes include prolonged PR interval, ST segment depression, T-wave flattening and the development of U waves. Mild degrees of preoperative hypokalaemia (down to 3.0 mmol/L) pose little perioperative risk to the patient who is otherwise well, and surgery should proceed in those circumstances. There is in fact little evidence that a K^+ of down to 2.6 mmol/L is associated with an increase in morbidity or mortality. If the patient is digitalised this threshold should obviously be raised.

The significance of hyperkalaemia rests with the risk of arrhythmias and cardiac arrest and our ability to produce it with intemperate use of suxamethonium. It is also seen in the reperfusion of ischaemic tissue, such as in crush injury. Both of these subjects are common scenarios in the exam. The ECG changes, which include prolonged PR interval, widening of the QRS and peaked T waves as a precursor to VF, are common exam fare. It should be treated if the K$^+$ is >6.5 mmol/L or ECG changes are present. The emergency management includes the combination of insulin and glucose, calcium and bicarbonate.

Chloride (Cl$^-$)

Chloride is the predominant extracellular anion (RR 100–110 mmol/L) and its distribution across the cell membrane follows the electro-chemical gradient as predicted by the Nernst equation. Derangements in chloride physiology are important, in that they are associated with disturbances in acid-base physiology. This is primarily the result of a bicarbonate–chloride exchange within the renal collecting tubule.

Hyperchloraemia may be seen as a result of dehydration, or as a consequence of metabolic acidosis or compensated respiratory alkalosis. The common scenario seen in anaesthesia practice is the patient who has been resuscitated with a large volume of 0.9% sodium chloride. This results in a non-anion gap metabolic acidosis, and the picture provides a nice blood gas for interpretation.

Hypochloraemia is seen with a range of disorders, including Addison's disease, gastric outlet obstruction, nasogastric suctioning, metabolic alkalosis, chronic compensated respiratory acidosis and congestive cardiac failure. The classic scenario for the anaesthetist is the child with pyloric stenosis, in which the child develops dehydration as a result of gastric outlet obstruction. The electrolytes show a hypochloraemic, hypokalaemic alkalosis. The candidate requires a good understanding of the mechanism of the metabolic derangement, a clear plan for its correction, and a threshold at which they would undertake surgery.

Bicarbonate (HCO$_3^-$)

The measurement of the serum bicarbonate is most frequently associated with the assessment of arterial blood gases. In the standard set of U&Es the measurement is obtained as a total CO_2 measured by spectrophotometry. This differs from the derived parameter recorded on a blood gas analysis. The bicarbonate buffer system holds great importance, in that the system allows control via respiratory and renal mechanisms to maintain pH. The normal range is 22–32 mmol/L.

Serum bicarbonate is elevated in metabolic alkalosis and compensated respiratory acidosis, and is decreased in metabolic acidosis. It is most likely to require comment as part of a blood gas assessment in the exam. However, an abnormal result on a set of U&Es should make you consider the underlying process (such as elevation in the CO_2 retainer). It may also be the guide to management in some clinical situations where a blood gas is not warranted, such as pyloric stenosis.

Calcium (Ca^{++})

Calcium is present in the blood in three forms, namely ionised, protein bound and complexed (chelated with phosphate, sulphate and citrate), and can be quantified as the total, ionised and corrected calcium. The total calcium is measured by spectrophotometry and the ionised by an ion-selective electrode. The corrected calcium is derived from a correction algorithm, correcting for the albumin level in an attempt to better reflect the physiological action of calcium.

The principal control of extracellular calcium is via the action of parathyroid hormone, which acts directly on bone and kidney and indirectly on the intestine (via vitamin D synthesis) to elevate the calcium concentration.

The reference ranges are:
- Total calcium   2.10–2.55 mmol/L
- Corrected calcium   2.15–2.55 mmol/L
- Ionised calcium   1.20–1.30 mmol/L

Hypocalcaemia in the perioperative patient is most commonly seen in the setting of a low albumin (burns, critical illness, etc), but the ionised calcium is usually normal. Acute hypoparathyroidism following surgical resection, rapid infusion of citrated blood and acute hyperventilation will decrease the ionised calcium.

Hypercalcaemia in the perioperative patient (and hence, exam scenario) is usually related to hyperparathyroidism (primary or secondary), sarcoidosis or other granulomatous disease, and malignancy. The clinical manifestations include mental state changes, vomiting and renal failure. Cardiac conduction changes include prolonged PR and QT intervals and widening of the QRS complex. Management generally involves diuretics, saline and steroids.

Urea and creatinine

Serum urea (RR 3.0–8.0 mmol/L) is measured because it is excreted by the kidney, and is therefore useful for the investigation of renal function. The level of urea increases because of decreased excretion due to decreased glomerular filtration seen in renal and pre-renal disease, and because of increased production states such as gastrointestinal bleeding.

Decreased serum urea is seen in pregnancy with water retention, and in situations of decreased production, such as severe liver disease.

Creatinine is produced by the breakdown of creatine phosphate in muscle at a relatively constant rate depending on the muscle mass. It is largely excreted unchanged by the kidney, and as it undergoes minimal tubular reabsorption the level can be used as a surrogate for glomerular filtration. The serum creatinine (reference range: 40–120 micromol/L, depending on age and sex) may be used to derive an estimate of the creatinine clearance via the Cockcroft and Gault formula. This estimate relies on the age, weight, sex and serum creatinine. The estimated glomerular filtration rate recorded on a standard U&E report does not correct for body size and is less accurate for the purposes of drug dosing, where this is critical.

The urea/creatinine ratio is used as an attempt to exploit the different mechanisms that change the levels of urea and creatinine. The values can be confusing due to the different units on offer, but the range should be provided in the exam situation. Elevation of the ratio generally points to pre-renal issues such as dehydration/hypovolaemia, or to gastrointestinal bleeding. A low value will tend to indicate intrinsic renal disease or the presence of a condition that leads to cause a low urea.

TABLE 6.23 Classic patterns of electrolyte abnormality

Condition	Electrolyte abnormality
Hyperadrenalism	• Hypernatraemia
	• Hypokalaemia
	• Metabolic alkalosis
Hypoadrenalism (Addison's syndrome)	• Hypo-osmolar hyponatraemia
	• Hyperkalaemia
	• Mildly increased urea
	• Mildly metabolic acidosis
	• Hypercalcaemia
Pyloric stenosis	• Hypokalaemia
	• Hypochloraemia
	• Metabolic alkalosis
	• Increased urea, variable creatinine
Beta adrenergic stimulation	• Lactic acidosis
	• Hypokalaemia
Excessive 0.9% saline administration	• Hyperchloraemia
	• Metabolic acidosis
	• Normal anion gap
Rhabdomyolysis	• Hyperkalaemia
	• Hyperphosphataemia
	• Hypocalcaemia
	• Increased CK

11. Respiratory function tests

Preoperative testing of pulmonary function in patients with suspected lung disease is common, and candidates should be familiar with frequently encountered abnormalities and patterns of results. Respiratory function tests are particularly useful in following individual patients over time, so comparison with previous results may be helpful. Candidates should also anticipate questions on respiratory function tests in association with other modalities of investigation, for example, chest X-ray or CT scan, and arterial blood gas analysis. Combinations of investigations in association with the clinical history and examination are most useful in yielding a definitive diagnosis and management plan.

For the purposes of the exam, candidates should be mindful of typical patterns obtained for obstructive, restrictive and mixed respiratory defects, and also of flow–volume patterns typical of fixed and variable (intra- and extra-thoracic) upper airway obstruction.

Spirometry

Simple spirometry from a standard bellows spirometer produces a volume vs time curve with the expired volume deflected upwards. Where several scales of measurement are present results should be recorded at body temperature and pressure saturated with water vapour (BTPS). The best recorded result from three maximal forceful expiratory attempts should be recorded, and expiratory time should be at least 6 seconds (Fig 6.56). Interpretation of results is based on a comparison with reference values of subjects matched for age, gender, height and ethnic origin. Traditionally, values >15% away from predicted values are considered abnormal.

Simple spirometry yields the following useful parameters:
- Forced expired volume in 1 second: FEV_1
- Forced vital capacity: FVC
- Ratio of FEV_1/FVC (expressed as a percentage): FEV_1/FVC %
- Forced expiratory flow over the middle half of the FVC (reflecting moderate to small airways): $FEF_{25-75\%}$
- Peak flow (PEF) measurement is the maximal expiratory flow rate achieved (hence the steepest gradient on a simple spirometer curve) and can also be measured by stand-alone portable devices. Such devices may have limited accuracy, but are useful for following trends in lung function for individual patients.

A reduction of FEV_1 relative to FVC is typical of obstructive defects (such as chronic bronchitis, emphysema and asthma) (Fig 6.57). FEV_1 is 60–80% predicted in mild disease, 40–59% predicted in moderate disease and <40% predicted in severe disease (British Thoracic Society Guidelines). Note that with early airways closure in obstructive airways disease the FVC may be underestimated by simple spirometry, leading to an overestimation of the $FEV_1/FVC\%$.

Restrictive defects (e.g. chest wall deformities, muscle weakness or interstitial lung disease) display a reduction in both FEV_1 and FVC, such that the $FEV_1/FVC\%$ remains normal or high (i.e. the reduction in FVC exceeds that of FEV_1) (Fig 6.58).

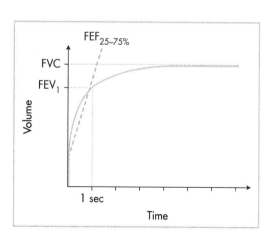

FIGURE 6.56 **Normal spirometry**

Occasionally a combination of both airway obstruction and restriction may be present, leading to a low $FEV_1/FVC\%$ in association with a markedly reduced FVC (Fig 6.59).

Reversibility of airway obstruction

Especially in asthma, the degree of reversibility of airflow obstruction can be quantified by the percentage improvement in FEV_1 15 minutes after the administration of a bronchodilator. While not universally accepted, a figure of

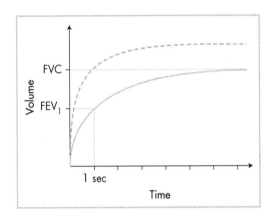

FIGURE 6.57 **Spirometry in obstructive lung disease**

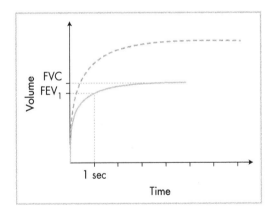

FIGURE 6.58 **Spirometry in restrictive lung disease**

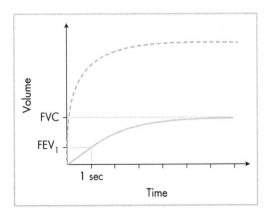

FIGURE 6.59 **Spirometry in mixed pulmonary disease**

12% improvement and an absolute improvement of >0.2 L may be considered significant. Note that an absence of improvement does not exclude a diagnosis of asthma as inflammatory processes may dominate in the absence of increased smooth muscle tone.

Flow–volume loops

Flow-sensing spirometers measure flow as the primary parameter and can digitally integrate the signal to produce a curve representing flow versus volume. Maximal inspiratory and expiratory flow curves produce characteristic appearances in health and disease (Figs 6.60–6.65).

Inspiratory flow rates in obstructive disease are usually minimally affected. There is a reduction in expiratory flow rates, and the curve typically has a concave or scalloped appearance. If significant air trapping is present both total lung capacity and residual volume will be increased, thus the flow–volume loop has a relative leftwards displacement on the X-axis (Fig 6.61).

The shape of the flow-volume loop in restrictive disease will demonstrate reduction of both total lung capacity and residual volume. Expiratory flows may be increased relative to lung volume. A steepness in the curve may reflect an increase in mid-expiratory flows caused by increased elastic recoil, and the curve typically has a convex appearance (Fig 6.62).

In diseases such as tracheal stenosis, lung volumes are unchanged, but there is constant reduction in both inspiratory and expiratory flows that cannot be

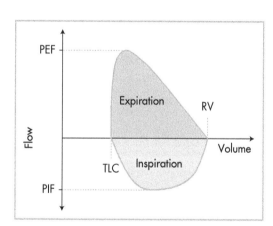

FIGURE 6.60 Normal flow–volume loop

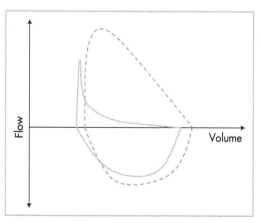

FIGURE 6.61 Flow–volume loop in obstructive lung disease

overcome by patient effort, leading to a characteristic flattened flow–volume curve (Fig 6.63).

In conditions such as vocal cord paralysis, inspiratory flow may be markedly reduced, with preservation of expiratory flow rates (Fig 6.64).

In contrast, lesions of the lower trachea may limit expiratory flow, but have little effect on airflow rates during inspiration (Fig 6.65).

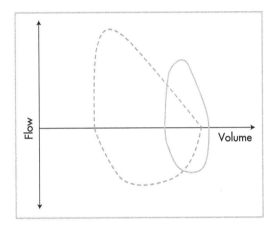

FIGURE 6.62 **Flow–volume loop in restrictive lung disease**

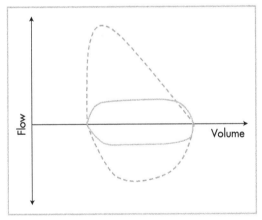

FIGURE 6.63 **Flow–volume loop with fixed upper airway obstruction**

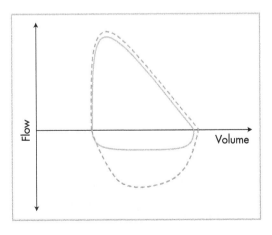

FIGURE 6.64 **Flow–volume loop with variable extrathoracic upper airway obstruction**

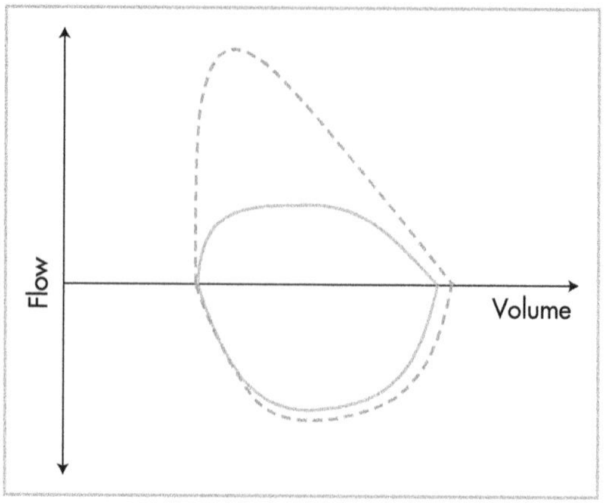

FIGURE 6.65 **Flow–volume loop with variable intrathoracic upper airway obstruction**

DLCO diffusion studies

For patients with undifferentiated dyspnoea, measuring the diffusion capacity of carbon monoxide (DLCO) may be of benefit. The test assesses transfer of gas by diffusion from alveoli to pulmonary capillaries, and relies on the strong affinity and large absorption capacity of erythrocytes for carbon monoxide. A low concentration (0.3%) of CO is inspired, and the exhaled concentration is measured after a 10-second breath hold. DLCO is calculated from the partial pressure difference.

Average values are 20–30 mL CO transferred/minute breathhold/mmHg driving pressure, but vary with age, sex, weight and height. Causes of abnormalities are shown in Table 6.24.

TABLE 6.24 Causes of a decrease or an increase in DLCO	
Decrease	**Increase**
Interstitial lung disease	Exercise
Emphysema	High altitude
Pulmonary hypertension	Polycythaemia
Anaemia	Left to right cardiac shunt
Cardiac insufficiency	Pulmonary haemorrhage
Pulmonary thromboembolism	Asthma
Hypothermia	Morbid obesity
Hypothyroidism	Hyperthyroidism

12. Sleep studies

Sleep apnoea, both diagnosed and undiagnosed, is an increasingly common condition in patients presenting for surgery. As the condition has a number of serious complications as well as important implications for anaesthesia, the candidate presenting for the final exam would be expected to understand the basics of a sleep study. In addition, it is a common condition in the type of patients selected for the medical viva, who will be likely to have undergone investigation for their sleep apnoea.

The archetypical patient suffering from sleep apnoea is a middle-aged, overweight male who enjoys alcohol. There will usually be complaints from their sleeping partner of snoring (among other things) with episodes of apnoea. The patient will typically complain of poor, disturbed sleep, daytime somnolence and headache.

The sleep study

The standard polysomnography study monitors at least seven physiological parameters, including electroencephalogram (EEG), electro-oculogram (EOG), chin electromyogram (EMG), the ECG and monitors of airflow, respiratory effort and arterial oxygen saturation. Leg movement and patient position are often also recorded. Most of this information would be of interest for the sleep physician, but for the anaesthetist serves only to confuse and clutter the report.

Interpretation of the sleep study

The essential information that you need to establish from the sleep study is:
- the nature of the sleep apnoea (central, obstructive or mixed); and
- the severity of the sleep apnoea.

This information then needs to be related to the clinical state of the patient.

The real-life study will come with an easy-to-interpret summary that illustrates the key findings. However, you may be presented with a bewildering set of numbers, abbreviations and graphs that you must quickly make some sense of. This means that you need to be able to select the important numbers from the mass of information in the body of the report. An example of standard sleep study data is presented in Table 6.25.

The study in Table 6.25 and Figure 6.66 provides an example of a patient with severe obstructive sleep apnoea. An apnoea in an adult is defined as the cessation of airflow for 10 or more seconds. The apnoea is termed obstructive if it is associated with discernable respiratory effort, and central if it is not. Just as important is the occurrence of a hypopnoea as it has the same pathological significance. The definitions vary, but it involves a respiratory event lasting at least 10 seconds with at least 4% fall in oxygen saturation and at least a 30% fall in

TABLE 6.25 Polysomnography report – statistics

Sleep statistics		
Report time: 21:41:55 to 05:16:54 = 455.0 min	Total sleep time:	194.5 min
Sleep latency = 36.5 min	NREM sleep = 171.0 min	87.9%
REM latency = 332.5 min	Stage 1 = 30.5 min	15.7%
	Stage 2 = 135.5 min	69.7%
Total time awake during	Stage 3 = 4.5 min	2.3%
sleep period = 220.0 min	Stage 4 = 0.5 min	0.3%
	REM sleep = 23.5 min	12.1%
Sleep efficiency: = 42.7%		

TABLE 6.25 Polysomnography report – statistics (cont'd)

Respiratory statistics

	NREM			REM		
	Back	Other	All	Back	Other	All
SpO_2% lowest:	87	71	71	–	57	57

RDI

Central apnoea	0.0	0.0	0.0	0.0	0.0	0.0
Obstructive apnoea	0.0	61.9	61.8	0.0	58.7	58.7
Hypopnoea	0.0	28.5	28.4	0.0	5.1	5.1
Apnoea+hypopnoea	0.0	90.4	90.2	0.0	63.8	63.8
TOTAL RDI			90.2			63.8

TOTAL RDI (REM + NREM) = 87.0

Longest apnoea = 85.0 sec

Longest hypopnoea = 58.1 sec

Mean apnoea/hypopnoea duration = 30.2 sec

Desaturation statistics

SpO_2% awake average =	91%	*Desaturation:*	*Number of:*
Nadir SpO_2% =	57%	≥ 2%	266
Average SpO_2 desaturation =	10%	≥3%	266
Average SpO_2% min (sleep time) =	81%	≥4%	260
%total sleep SpO_2<90% =	69.2%	≥5%	251

%total sleep SpO_2<80% =17.0%

Arousal statistics (sleep time)

Number of:	REM	NREM	Total	Per hour:	REM	NREM	Total
ORE	0	0	0	ORE	0.0	0.0	0.0
CRE	0	0	0	CRE	0.0	0.0	0.0
ORE	22	266	288	ORE	56.2	93.3	88.8
Unsure	0	4	4	Unsure	0.0	1.4	1.2
PLM	0	0	0	PLM	0.0	0.0	0.0
			292	Arousal index:			90.1

Heart rate statistics

Maximum heart rate (report time):	247 beats/min
Minimum heart rate (report time):	12 beats/min
Average heart rate (report time):	57 beats/min

Leg movement statistics

PLM per hour of sleep:	0.0
PLM per hour of NREM sleep:	0.0
PLM per hour of REM sleep:	0.0

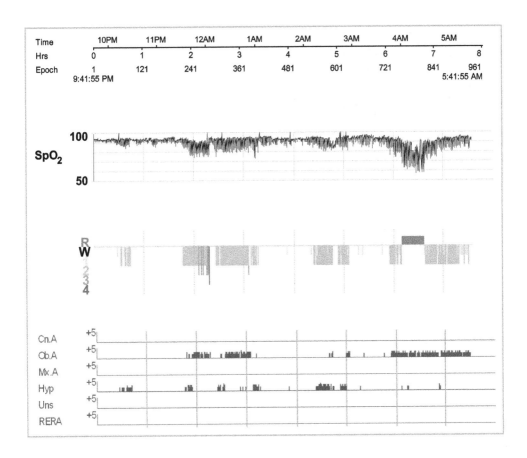

FIGURE 6.66 **Polysomnography report – graphical**

airflow compared to baseline. Related to hypopnoeas is the Respiratory Effort Related Arousal (RERA), which are obstructive events that lead to arousal from sleep. They are on the bottom graph (there are none present in the case above).

Probably the most useful number to be produced is the apnoea hypopnoea index (AHI) or the respiratory disturbance index (RDI), which is quoted in the case above. The AHI is the number of respiratory events (apnoeas and hypopnoeas) recorded per hour of sleep. Obstructive sleep apnoea is defined as mild if the AHI is 5–15, moderate if 16–30, and severe if it is >30. The RDI adds in the RERAs, but the severity definitions are essentially the same.

The respiratory statistics will also separate the apnoeas into central, obstructive and mixed. This study indicates, with both tables and graphs, that the apnoeas are all of an obstructive nature. To diagnose obstructive sleep apnoea, more than 75% of the apnoeas or hypopnoeas must have an obstructive pattern. There are also multiple arousals and desaturations. The arousal index is the number of arousals per hour of sleep, where there is EEG evidence that the patient has moved to a lighter plane of sleep.

If the patient has significant sleep apnoea, you need to consider associated complications such as pulmonary hypertension and right ventricular changes, systemic hypertension, congestive cardiac failure, and respiratory failure with

CO_2 retention. Anticipate being shown further investigations, such as ECGs and echocardiograph results, in this situation.

If the patient has central sleep apnoea the apnoea episode is related to the periodic loss of respiratory drive. These may be idiopathic, but often relates to disease states such as congestive heart failure, cerebrovascular accident, thyroid disease or opioid medication.

Answers to data interpretation cases

Electrocardiography

Case 1
  a The first ECG (Fig 6.1) demonstrates a tachycardia of approximately 170 beats per minute. The QRS complexes appear slightly widened with an RSR' pattern present in many leads.

  b The differential diagnosis might include ventricular tachycardia or supraventricular tachycardia.

  c Immediate treatment would include monitoring of other vital signs (including blood pressure and pulse oximetry), establishment of intravenous access and oxygen administration. This patient was diagnosed with a supraventricular tachycardia, and treated successfully with intravenous adenosine.

  d The second trace (Fig 6.2) demonstrates normal sinus rhythm of 60 beats per minute, with characteristic delta wave shortening of the PR interval, consistent with a diagnosis of Wolff-Parkinson-White syndrome. The significance of the Q waves in the inferior leads is unclear.

Case 2
  a The ECG in Figure 6.3 shows large amplitude QRS complexes in the praecordial leads with ST depression evident in the lateral leads. These findings are consistent with left ventricular hypertrophy and ventricular strain pattern, in keeping with the diagnosis of severe aortic stenosis suggested by the history and examination findings.

  b Further appropriate investigations would include chest X-ray and echocardiography.

Case 3
  a The ECG in Figure 6.4 is characterised by first degree heart block (prolonged PR interval), right bundle branch block (RSR' pattern in anterior leads) and left anterior hemi block (left axis deviation).

  b Thus the patient has a tri-fascicular block and is at increased risk of complete heart block, severe bradyarrhythmias and sudden cardiac death. He should be referred urgently for consideration for insertion of a permanent pacemaker prior to undertaking any elective surgery.

Case 4
  a Early sections of the ECG in Figure 6.5 show pacing spikes and ST elevation consistent with an acute inferior myocardial infarct. As the trace is taken a wide-complex tachycardia ensues (which in lead V4 appears to have some features consistent with torsades de pointes), which further degenerates into ventricular fibrillation in the rhythm strip taken as lead II.

  b This is a medical emergency. Appropriate cardiopulmonary resuscitative measures (including defibrillation) should be immediately instigated.

Case 5 a Sudden onset of chest pain after major surgery should alert the clinician to several possibilities, including myocardial ischaemia, pulmonary atelectasis and/or infection and pulmonary thromboembolism.

             b The ECG in Figure 6.6 shows anterior lead T-wave inversion, small S waves in lead I, Q waves in lead III and T-wave inversion in lead III (S1Q3T3 pattern suggestive of acute cor pulmonale), all of which are consistent with a diagnosis of pulmonary embolism (other common ECG findings are tachycardia and right bundle branch block). It should be kept in mind that the ECG is in itself a poor diagnostic test for pulmonary embolism, but useful in ruling out myocardial ischaemia in the patient with sudden onset chest pain.

             c Further investigations might include CT pulmonary angiography or ventilation/perfusion scanning.

Case 6 a This patient was suffering from severe hyperkalaemia secondary to acute rhabdomyolysis. The ECG in Figure 6.7 shows a broadening of the QRS complexes and peaked T waves in the praecordium, with T-wave inversion inferiorly. The serum potassium was 7.0 mmol/L.

             b Shortly thereafter (Fig 6.8), the serum potassium was 8.9 mmol/L, and the ECG demonstrates further QRS widening with a sinusoidal appearance; such a development may have been precipitated by administration of suxamethonium.

             c Rapid measures must be undertaken to prevent ventricular standstill (e.g. oxygen administration, airway and ventilatory support, calcium gluconate, insulin/dextrose infusions, bicarbonate, dialysis).

Case 7 a The ECG in Figure 6.9 has an unusual appearance; there is a predominance of S waves in QRS complexes with virtually no R wave progression across the ECG. P wave inversion is present in lead I, which, in the absence of incorrectly applied ECG leads, suggests a diagnosis of dextrocardia.

             b Isolated dextrocardia should be differentiated from complete situs inversus, as other developmental anomalies and complications differ between the two groups. Chest X-ray and CT scanning would be appropriate before further advice is given.

Case 8 a The ECG in Figure 6.10 demonstrates marked sinus arrhythmia.

             b This finding is common in children, as is the presence of an innocent ejection systolic murmur.

             c In an otherwise healthy child there is generally no need to postpone surgery; further investigation can be carried out electively in an outpatient setting.

Case 9 a The ECG in Figure 6.11 shows a ventricular rate of 35 beats per minute. P waves are present, but only every second P wave is followed by a QRS complex, i.e. there is second degree atrioventricular block (Mobitz type II).

             b This represents disease of the His-Purkinje system and may rapidly progress to complete heart block. This patient requires urgent referral for permanent pacing.

Case 10 a The characteristic saw-tooth appearance of atrial flutter (in this case with variable AV block) is best demonstrated in the rhythm strip of Figure 6.12.

b The rhythm is usually unstable and may degenerate into atrial fibrillation. Persistent atrial flutter tends to be resistant to cardioversion, but the abnormal pathway may be ablated electrophysiologically.

Case 11 a The ECG in Figure 6.13 shows a broad-complex tachycardia with a ventricular rate of 150 beats per minute. The most common diagnostic dilemma is to differentiate ventricular tachycardia from supraventricular tachycardia with aberrant conduction.

b Criteria established by Brugada suggest that a diagnosis of VT is more likely with an absence of an RS complex in all praecordial leads, R to S interval (when present) greater than 100 ms, when atrioventricular dissociation is present and with characteristic morphology patterns in leads V1 and V6 when a notched ventricular complex is present.

c In this instance, the diagnosis was ventricular tachycardia. Note that amiodarone can usually be used safely in either eventuality. Further electrophysiological studies are indicated.

Case 12 a The ECG in Figure 6.14 demonstrates some features of a true posterior myocardial infarct.

b Changes are 'mirrored' in the anterior chest leads, i.e. instead of a Q wave, there is a tall R wave, ST depression rather than elevation is seen, and an upright T wave is present. It is common for other areas of the heart to be involved, and there is a suggestion of inferior ST elevation in this trace. Typical changes of infarction can be demonstrated with more posterior chest leads (e.g. V7, V8, V9).

c Aside from usual resuscitative measures, further management depends on the availability of angioplasty or thrombolysis.

Case 13 a The common side effect of all three medications taken by this patient is prolongation of the QT interval, which is demonstrated in Figure 6.15. As the QT interval is rate dependent, the corrected QT interval (QTc) should be calculated: $QTc = QT/\sqrt{R{-}R}$. In this case the QT interval is 0.38 sec and the heart rate is approximately 120 beats/min (so the R–R interval is 0.5 sec). $QTc = 0.38/\sqrt{0.5} = 0.54$. This is markedly prolonged (normal QTc $\leq$ 0.44) and predisposes the patient to R on T phenomena including torsades de pointes and other ventricular arrhythmias.

b Electrolyte abnormalities and congenital QT syndrome are other possible causes.

Case 14 a Figure 6.16 shows widespread saddle-shaped ST segment elevation, and areas of PR segment depression, both of which are characteristic of acute pericarditis.

Chest radiography

Case 15 a Figure 6.28 shows obvious mirror image reversal of the cardiac shadow (dextrocardia) with other features of complete situs inversus: the left hemidiaphragm is higher than the right (implying underlying liver), gastric bubble is present on the right side and a wider, more vertical left main bronchus is seen on the left side.

b Patients with complete situs inversus may have no other medical problems, but associated abnormalities should be excluded. CT scanning is appropriate and ECG clinically interesting.

Case 16 a The X-ray in Figure 6.29 shows blunting of both costophrenic angles, consistent with a diagnosis of bilateral pleural effusion.

Case 17 a The X-ray in Figure 6.30 shows an endotracheal tube, ECG electrodes and leads, oro- or naso-gastric tube and left subclavian central venous line (the tip of which is probably in the right atrium).

b The increased opacification centrally on the lung fields is non-expanded lung tissue. There are large bilateral pneumothoraces (keep in mind that this is a supine film) with deepening of both costophrenic angles (deep sulcus sign). Urgent drainage is required.

Case 18 a Figure 6.31 demonstrates complete opacification of the left hemithorax with mediastinal shift to the left side. This is almost certainly due to complete left lung collapse caused by right endobronchial intubation.

b On examination, the patient would have asymmetric chest movement, left tracheal deviation and decreased or absent breath sounds on the left side.

Case 19 a Figure 6.32 is a supine mobile film. There is an endotracheal tube, left internal jugular central venous line and ECG electrodes and leads. There are multiple lateral and posterior rib fractures (this patient in fact had a flail chest) and left-sided pulmonary contusion (accounting for the difference in lung field opacification between the two sides).

Case 20 a Surgical clips from the recent operation are visible in the right upper quadrant of the abdomen. However, the main abnormality in Figure 6.33 is a marked widening of the mediastinum, with an opacification which appears to be continuous with the aorta; in this case a massively dilated thoracic aortic aneurysm secondary to atherosclerosis. Calcification can be seen in its wall, and there is some compression and rightward displacement of the trachea.

b Contrast CT scanning is probably the most useful imaging modality to further evaluate the lesion, and the patient requires significant medical work-up if major thoracic surgery is to be undertaken.

Echocardiography

Case 21   a   Table 6.8 shows this patient has severe calcific aortic stenosis, with left ventricular hypertrophy, mild to moderate pulmonary hypertension and pseudo-normal diastolic dysfunction (there is raised left atrial pressure).

     b   A commonly encountered exam question. You should have some well-reasoned arguments. This patient may be able to be managed conservatively. Spinal anaesthesia should be avoided. An opioid-based general anaesthesia with invasive monitoring is feasible.

Case 22   a   This patient has dilated cardiomyopathy with severe systolic failure and a restrictive diastolic failure pattern (Table 6.9). The left atrium is dilated. Mitral regurgitation is probably secondary to ventricular dilatation. There is mild pulmonary hypertension. There are regional wall motion abnormalities in keeping with infarction in the territory of the left anterior descending artery.

     b   Myocardial ischaemia from atheromatous coronary artery disease is the most likely cause. This is in keeping with evidence of regional wall motion abnormalities.

Case 23   a   This patient has severe mitral stenosis with a dilated left atrium and pulmonary hypertension (Table 6.10).

     b   Such cases are almost invariably secondary to rheumatic fever.

     c   One possible approach is epidural at term prior to onset of labour with gentle incremental top-ups and invasive monitoring. Generally patients with more severe disease, especially if severe pulmonary hypertension is present, should be delivered by caesarean section under general anaesthesia. If the patient presented in early pregnancy, consideration would need to be given to termination.

Case 24   a   This patient has severe aortic regurgitation with a dilated left ventricle and borderline hypertrophy (Table 6.11). The ventricular function is likely preserved, but the ejection fraction gives a falsely reassuring impression in the face of regurgitant lesions. There is dilatation of the aortic root.

     b   The patient is likely to require a Bentall procedure (composite graft replacement of the aortic valve, aortic root and ascending aorta, with re-implantation of the coronary arteries into the graft). Indications vary, but an aortic diameter of 5 cm and a valve that requires operation (the left ventricle is dilating) means that the surgeon would probably replace the aortic root as well as the valve.

Case 25   a   Pulmonary hypertension and right ventricular hypertrophy are present (Table 6.12). The left ventricle and valves appear normal.

     b   Based on the history, the most likely cause is primary pulmonary hypertension, but this is a diagnosis of exclusion. Other possible causes include chronic respiratory disease or hypoxia, thromboembolic disease, other inflammatory disease of pulmonary vasculature (e.g. sarcoid, collagen vascular diseases).

Case 26 a In Table 6.13 Qp:Qs is the ratio of relative cardiac output through the pulmonary and systemic circulations respectively.

b A ratio of 2:1 is the generally accepted indication for defect closure. The presence of symptoms of reversible pulmonary hypertension may prompt closure at lower shunts of around 1.5:1. The presence of a defect with a history of cerebrovascular accident may also prompt closure of a smaller defect.

Arterial blood gas analysis

Case 27 a This patient has diabetic ketoacidosis (DKA).

b Along with a suggestive history, there is marked hyperglycaemia and a high anion gap metabolic acidosis (Table 6.14).

c Although the serum potassium is high, there is usually overall total body depletion. Urinalysis is indicated.

d DKA is a medical emergency. Candidates should have a comprehensive management strategy for such a case, the detailing of which is beyond the scope of this book.

Case 28 a This patient has an acute respiratory alkalosis (Table 6.15). The metabolic compensation is as expected and there is no evidence of a mixed disorder.

b The most likely explanation in an otherwise well patient is inappropriate mechanical ventilation settings with excessive minute ventilation. Reduce the set tidal volume, respiratory rate, or both.

Case 29 a This patient has a mixed metabolic alkalosis and respiratory acidosis (Table 6.16). The pH is almost within the given reference range, but both the pCO_2 and HCO_3 are markedly elevated.

b The metabolic alkalosis is easily explained from loss of gastric acid. However, the pCO_2 is higher than would be expected for respiratory compensation of this degree of metabolic alkalosis. A respiratory acidosis therefore coexists, perhaps from central respiratory depression from opiate administration or pre-existing disease.

c Fluid replacement, taking into account intravascular volume status, intraoperative and ongoing losses, and potential electrolyte imbalances should be established.

Case 30 a The patient has a mixed respiratory and metabolic acidosis (Table 6.17). The respiratory acidosis is easily explained from the long-standing chronic pulmonary disease. With such a vague presentation the possible causes of metabolic acidosis in this patient are many.

b Initially, calculation of an anion gap will help to refine the differential diagnosis. Serum glucose, serum electrolytes, liver function tests, markers of cardiac injury and thyroid function tests may also help narrow the list of possible causes.

Coagulation studies

Case 31 a This is likely to be von Willebrand's disease (Table 6.18). Consult with a haematologist, who will measure platelet function, factor VIII activity and von Willebrand's factor. Traditionally they would have conducted a bleeding time in this circumstance (expect prolongation), but that is rarely done now. The subtype should also be characterised (most likely type I on the information provided).

b Most mild cases will respond to intravenous DDAVP, 0.3 mcg/kg.

Case 32 a The likely diagnosis in this case is amniotic fluid embolism (Table 6.19).

b The coagulopathy is caused by disseminated intravascular coagulation.

Case 33 a This patient is likely to have obstructive jaundice causing malabsorption of vitamin K (Table 6.20).

b Initial management options include intravenous vitamin K and fresh frozen plasma.

Case 34 a This patient has idiopathic thrombocytopaenic purpura, due to the development of antiplatelet antibodies (usually IgG) causing platelet destruction in the spleen (Table 6.21).

b Management should include steroids/IV immunoglobulin preoperatively to increase platelet count. The patient should be immunised against haemophilus influenzae B, pneumococcus and meningococcus. Platelet infusion prior to splenectomy is usually pointless.

Case 35 a This patient has liver failure (Table 6.22). The mechanism of the coagulation defect is multifactorial and includes failure of clotting factor synthesis, vitamin K deficiency and fibrinolysis. The fall in platelet count is probably the result of hypersplenism and bone marrow dysfunction. Portal hypertension causing oesophageal varices is the likely source of bleeding.

b The patient requires vitamin K and fresh frozen plasma. Red cell and platelet transfusion will probably also be required.

Chapter 7

Useful reference and review articles

Overview

Critical appraisal of the literature is a required skill of consultant anaesthetists, and increasingly candidates may be expected to provide informed scientific rationale to justify responses to questions in the final exam.

Papers relevant to anaesthetic practice are being published at an exponentially increasing rate. Wading through this enormous volume of knowledge to extract valuable information is more time-consuming and difficult than ever before.

For the purposes of the final examination much important knowledge can be gleaned from the many excellent review articles published in major journals, and candidates are wise to concentrate their reading on such papers. Many short answer examination questions appear to have been drawn directly from major reviews of a specific topic, familiarity with which can greatly enhance a candidate's ability to provide a detailed structured response.

Other papers that deserve special attention include large, multicentre trials which are likely to influence clinical practice (especially those originating in Australasia), comprehensive meta-analyses on important topics, and clinical trials that appear in well-respected non-anaesthetic journals (such as *The Lancet* and *The New England Journal of Medicine*). In recent years the written paper has also included questions related to the conduct of anaesthetic research, statistical methodology and topics requiring an understanding of current scientific opinion for a successful response.

This chapter lists articles on a wide range of topics that may be of interest to candidates. This list is not intended to be all-inclusive, and candidates are strongly urged to compile their own reference collection in preparation for the examination. Each entry is accompanied by a brief summary of its content.

Airway management and spinal injury

Crosby ET. Airway management in adults after cervical spine trauma. Anesthesiology 2006; 104:1293–318.

- A lengthy and comprehensive review of cervical spine injuries encompassing functional anatomy of the cervical spine and mechanisms of bony and spinal cord injuries. Epidemiological data and diagnostic dilemmas are addressed and options for securing the airway discussed, including an in-depth analysis of cervical spine movement with different techniques. The authors conclude that the majority of secondary neurological injuries are not a result of airway interventions, and they support the range of options currently accepted in clinical practice.

Ford P, Nolan J. Cervical spine injury and airway management. Curr Opin Anaesthesiol 2002; 15:193–201.
- This article discusses the difficulty in diagnosing cervical spine injuries in trauma patients, and discusses options for gaining control of the airway in such patients.

Hambly PR, Martin B. Anaesthesia for chronic spinal cord lesions. Anaesthesia 1998; 53:273–89.
- This review of the literature examines perioperative complications of longstanding spinal cord injuries, with an emphasis on autonomic dysreflexia and its prevention. The authors present a series of more than 500 cases. Although now somewhat dated, this still contains information of relevance for modern practice.

Henderson JJ, Popat MT, Latto IP, et al. Difficult Airway Society guidelines for management of the unanticipated difficult intubation. Anaesthesia 2004; 59:675–94.
- It would be unusual for a candidate not to be asked about their management of a difficult intubation in the examination. This article gives interesting insight into the development of guidelines and flowcharts for such situations. Descriptions of flowcharts for three situations are provided: difficult intubation at routine induction, difficult intubation during rapid sequence induction and failed intubation with increasing hypoxaemia and difficult ventilation in the paralysed patient. Guidelines for paediatric and obstetric patients are not provided.

Janssens M, Hartstein G. Management of difficult intubation. Eur J Anaesthesiol 2001; 18:3–12.
- An interesting essay on management of the difficult airway, including an anticipatory 'quantification scale'. Algorithms for anticipated/unexpected difficult intubation and failed intubation and failed ventilation scenarios are provided.

Mason RA, Fielder CP. The obstructed airway in head and neck surgery (editorial). Anaesthesia 1999; 54(7):625–8.
- A landmark editorial and essential reading. Discusses in detail the difficulties in decision-making and management when dealing with airway obstruction, and why awake fibre-optic bronchoscopy is not a universal panacea.

Pierre EJ, McNeer RR, Shamir MY. Early management of the traumatized airway. Anesthesiol Clin 2007; 25:1–11.
- A rational approach to the management of injuries to the airway, neck and face is presented, including the differences encountered in blunt vs penetrating injuries, and types of emergency surgical airways and the indications for these.

Stevens RD, Bhardwaj A, Kirsch JR, et al. Critical care and perioperative management in traumatic spinal cord injury. J Neurosurg Anesthesiol 2003; 15:215–29.

- This review discusses the epidemiology of spinal cord injury and its complications. It re-examines the controversies surrounding the efficacy of systemic steroids and other trials of pharmacological neuroprotection.

Allergy and anaphylaxis

Fisher MM, Baldo BA. Mast cell tryptase in anaesthetic anaphylactoid reactions. Br J Anaesth 1998; 80:26–9.

- The authors of this study collected serum for tryptase analysis in 350 patients after suspected anaphylactic reactions during anaesthesia. It was shown with concomitant intradermal testing and radioimmunoassay for serum antibodies that tryptase does not invariably rise during IgE mediated reactions, but nonetheless was a valuable indicator in the majority of patients. Tryptase does not always differentiate between anaphylactic and anaphylactoid reactions and may be an indicator of direct histamine release.

Hepner DL, Castells MC. Anaphylaxis during the perioperative period. Anesth Analg 2003; 97:1381–95.

- The authors review the pathophysiology and epidemiology of anaphylactic and anaphylactoid reactions related to anaesthesia. Muscle relaxants and latex are confirmed as the main culprits, but many other agents are discussed in detail. Diagnostic techniques including serum tryptase, skin prick, intradermal testing and advanced serology are described. Prevention and management of reactions are also covered.

Anaesthesia and co-existing disease

Adams JP, Murphy PG. Obesity in anaesthesia and intensive care. Br J Anaesth 2000; 85:91–108.

- This review article deals with the epidemiology of obesity and the pathophysiology of the associated cardiovascular and respiratory derangements. Practical anaesthetic considerations with regards to premedications, positioning, intravenous access, monitoring, regional techniques, analgesia and applied pharmacology are discussed.

Allen M. Pacemakers and implantable cardioverter defibrillators. Anaesthesia 2006; 61:883–90.

- This review provides candidates with a history of pacemaker development, pacemaker and defibrillator coding conventions and a description of pacing modes most frequently encountered. Perioperative patient management, causes of electromagnetic interference and the use of magnets are discussed in detail.

Avidan MS, Jones N, Pozniak AL. The implications of HIV for the anaesthetist and the intensivist. Anaesthesia 2000; 55:344–54.

- This is an excellent summary of the pathophysiology of HIV infection and deals with post-exposure prophylaxis and monitoring, antiretroviral agents and drug interactions, and co-morbidities of relevance to anaesthesia. Special attention is given to pain management in patients with HIV, and obstetrics and HIV.

Blasco LM, Parameshwar J, Vuysteke A. Anaesthesia for noncardiac surgery in the heart transplant recipient. Curr Opin Anaesthesiol 2009; 22:109–13.
- This recent review is a basic but easily read overview of issues faced by the cardiac transplant recipient, with sections on the physiology of the transplanted heart, complications following transplantation, immunosuppression and perioperative management.

Booker PD, Whyte SD, Ladusans EJ. Long QT syndrome and anaesthesia. Br J Anaesth 2003; 90:349–66.
- This review gives a comprehensive yet clearly explained account of the diagnostic criteria and genetic variants causing long QT syndrome, presented in the context of a detailed account of ion channel physiology. A useful list of drugs known to prolong the QT interval is provided, and perioperative patient management is discussed in detail, including the benefits of propofol-based anaesthesia and management of torsades de pointes, should it occur.

Byers J, Sladen RN. Renal function and dysfunction. Curr Opin Anaesthesiol 2001; 14:699–706.
- Evaluation of risks for renal dysfunction and controversies surrounding protective interventions are discussed, specifically in relation to cardiac surgery, aortic surgery and renal revascularisation. Risks associated with specific agents (including radiocontrast dye, volatile agents, cyclosporin, prostaglandin inhibitors) are discussed, as is renal transplantation.

Christ M, Sharkova Y, Geldner G, et al. Preoperative and perioperative care for patients with suspected or established aortic stenosis facing noncardiac surgery. Chest 2005; 128:2944–53.
- It would be unusual not to encounter questions on the management of aortic stenosis in the final examination. This article succinctly summarises cardiovascular risk in these patients and deals with preoperative risk assessment, including clinical assessment and echocardiographic findings. Intraoperative management principles are discussed only briefly, but the section on antibiotic prophylaxis is comprehensively tabulated.

Craig RG, Hunter JM. Recent developments in the perioperative management of adult patients with chronic kidney disease. Br J Anaesth 2008; 101:296–310.
- These authors provide a classification of chronic renal disease based on glomerular filtration rate (GFR), along with methods and equations for its estimation. Complications of chronic renal impairment and pharmacological hazards to this subgroup of patients are discussed, with an emphasis on fluid and electrolyte management. The article examines the use of general anaesthetic agents, neuromuscular blockers and analgesics in the setting of chronic kidney disease, including the use of agents such as sugammadex and remifentanil. Complications of commonly used immunosuppressants (in post-transplant patients) are briefly mentioned.

Croinyn DF, Shorten GD. Anesthesia and renal disease. Curr Opin Anaesthesiol 2002; 15:359–63.
- This review deals with the following current issues in the perioperative management of patients with renal disease: use of sevoflurane at low, fresh gas flow rates, endovascular vs open aortic aneurysm repair and postoperative renal function, use of thoracic epidural analgesia for cardiac surgery in renal patients, and the concomitant use of ketorolac and sevoflurane on renal function.

Dorotta IR, Schubert A. Multiple sclerosis and anesthetic implications. Curr Opin Anaesthesiol 2002; 15:365–70.
- The pathophysiology and clinical course of multiple sclerosis is discussed, as are the respiratory, autonomic and pharmacological implications for anaesthesia in these patients. Problems with neuromuscular blockade, regional techniques and temperature management of MS sufferers are also examined.

Fischer LG, Van Aken H, Buerkle H. Management of pulmonary hypertension: physiological and pharmacological considerations for anesthesiologists. Anesth Analg 2003; 96:1603–16.
- This article is a concise, very useful overview for those interested in the pulmonary circulation. Anatomy and physiology are well summarised in two pages, and the pathophysiology of pulmonary hypertension is discussed, including a consideration of mechanisms of vascular remodelling. The role of the right ventricle is given suitable emphasis. Causes of pulmonary hypertension are listed, including those encountered during anaesthesia (such as emboli, bone cement and extracorporeal circulation). Therapeutic management options are discussed, along with anaesthetic strategies for dealing with these patients.

Gross JB, Bachenberg KL, Benumof JL, et al. Practice guidelines for the perioperative management of patients with obstructive sleep apnea: a report by the American Society of Anesthesiologists task force on perioperative management of patients with obstructive sleep apnea. Anesthesiology 2006; 104(5):1081–93.
- This is an extensive set of consensus guidelines by the ASA for the management of these patients. The paper is well structured with fairly clear recommendations, along with some useful tables.

Hirsch NP, Murphy A, Radcliffe JJ. Neurofibromatosis: clinical presentations and anaesthetic implications. Br J Anaesth 2001; 86:555–64.
- A comprehensive discussion of the genetics and pathophysiology of neurofibromatosis, including cardiorespiratory complications. Features of the disease of relevance to the anaesthetist are highlighted.

Hodges PJ, Kam PCA. The perioperative implications of herbal medicines. Anaesthesia 2002; 57:889–99.
- This review documents the fact that a large proportion of patients may be taking herbal preparations that may interfere with anaesthesia, and that the majority of patients will not voluntarily reveal this fact. The pharmacologic implications of echinacea, garlic, ephedra, ginkgo, ginseng, kava, St John's Wort, valerian, ginger and grapefruit juice are specifically examined. The specific influence of

preparations on cardiovascular effect, coagulation, drug interactions (including prolongation of anaesthesia) and adverse immunological effects is discussed.

Huffmyer JL, Littlewood KE, Nemergut EC. Perioperative management of the adult with cystic fibrosis. Anesth Analg 2009; 109:1949–61.
- This review highlights the fact that cystic fibrosis patients are now living well into adulthood and are therefore more likely to require anaesthesia and surgery in adult hospitals. The effects of the condition on multiple organs and perioperative management are discussed in detail. The special considerations of lung and liver transplantation, and pregnancy are also discussed.

Isono S. Obstructive sleep apnea in obese adults: pathophysiology and perioperative airway management. Anesthesiology 2009; 110(4):908–21.
- This paper outlines the pathophysiology of obstructive sleep apnoea and its relationship to obesity in some detail. The author then presents personal views regarding the perioperative management of these patients, including a useful table regarding where and how to manage them postoperatively.

James MF, Hift RJ. Porphyrias. Br J Anaesth 2000; 85(1):143–53.
- A concise review of porphyrin metabolism and classification of the porphyrias. The authors detail the identification of susceptible individuals, tabulate recommendations on the use of an extensive list of anaesthetic drugs, and detail a course of action if a susceptible individual is administered a potentially triggering agent.

Jensen NF, Fiddler DS, Striepe V. Anesthetic considerations in porphyrias. Anesth Analg 1995; 80:591–9.
- Porphyrias are a rare but anaesthetically interesting group of disorders. In particular, anaesthetists should have an understanding of the pathophysiology, classification and symptomatology of the various enzyme defects in porphyrias, and a knowledge of which pharmacological agents to avoid. All of this information is well documented in this somewhat dated review, along with a useful summary of perioperative management strategies for dealing with affected patients.

Keegan MT, Plevak DJ. The transplant recipient for nontransplant surgery. Anaesthesiology Clin N Amer 2004; 22:827–61.
- An extensive review of the implications of anaesthesia on the transplant recipient. The paper has specific sections on lung, heart, liver, kidney, pancreas, intestinal and stem cell transplant. Each section outlines the anaesthetic concerns specific to each type of transplant, making the information easily accessible.

Kostopanagiotou G, Smyrniotis V, Arkadopoulos N, et al. Anesthetic and perioperative management of adult transplant recipients in nontransplant surgery. Anesth Analg 1999; 89:613–22.
- It is increasingly common to encounter transplant recipients in everyday situations. This article provides a good summary of the effects and hazards (including pharmacological interactions) of commonly used immunosuppressive agents. It also discusses perioperative management of transplant patients, including specific concerns for recipients of kidney, liver, heart, lung, pancreas and intestinal grafts. It deals with specific problems posed by trauma, pregnancy and laparoscopic surgery.

Loadsman JA, Hillman DR. Anaesthesia and sleep apnoea. Br J Anaesth 2001; 86:254–66.
- This review discusses the pathophysiology of obstructive sleep apnoea, symptoms, signs and sequelae of the disease. Specific perioperative risks and treatment options are presented.

Macarthur A, Kleiman S. Rheumatoid cervical joint disease – a challenge to the anaesthetist. Can J Anaesth 1993; 40:154–9.
- This article describes the various anatomical derangements that can occur in the cervical spine of patients with severe rheumatoid arthritis, including a subclassification of atlanto-axial subluxation. Use of radiology to predict the most appropriate positioning of patients to avoid further injury is discussed.

Nicholson G, Pereira AC, Hall GM. Parkinson's disease and anaesthesia. Br J Anaesth 2002; 89:904–16.
- This review provides a concise account of the pathophysiology of Parkinson's disease, including relevant neuroanatomy and motor pathways. The synopsis of clinical features of the disease is comprehensive. The authors then consider specific cardiovascular, gastrointestinal and autonomic abnormalities of particular anaesthetic interest, along with a brief consideration of the effects of common anaesthetic agents on patients with the condition.

Petroni KC, Cohen NH. Continuous renal replacement therapy: anesthetic implications. Anesth Analg 2002; 94:1288–97.
- This detailed article discusses the mechanisms of the different forms of continuous renal replacement therapy and compares them to the more conventional intermittent peritoneal and haemodialysis techniques, including indications for each. Preoperative assessment and intraoperative management of patients is discussed, along with the anaesthetic implications of such therapy.

Salukhe TV, Dob D, Sutton R. Pacemakers and defibrillators: anaesthetic implications. Br J Anaesth 2004; 93:95–104.
- This is another good review of pacemakers and defibrillators, outlining the basic physiology of cardiac pacing, problems with electromagnetic interference, pacemaker programming, use of magnets and an approach to patient evaluation and perioperative care.

Skues MA, Welchew EA. Anaesthesia and rheumatoid arthritis. Anaesthesia 1993; 48:989–97.
- This more dated review of anaesthesia for patients with rheumatoid arthritis still carries great relevance today. Preoperative assessment for articular and systemic manifestations, drug disposition and airway management are discussed in detail.

Stierer TS, Punjabi NM. Demographics and diagnosis of obstructive sleep apnea. Anesthesiol Clin N Amer 2005; 23:405–20.
- These authors provide good definitions of patterns of disordered breathing in sleep apnoea, along with several polysomnographic examples. They discuss

risk factors in turn (obesity, gender, age, race, craniofacial abnormalities, family history and alcohol consumption).

Toller WG, Metzler H. Acute perioperative heart failure. Curr Opin Anaesthesiol 2005; 18:129–35.
- This is a reasonable review of the mechanisms, diagnosis and management of conditions causing acute heart failure, including a succinct overview of the biochemical mechanisms underlying these disorders and their diagnosis and pharmacological treatments. The role of B-natriuretic peptide testing is discussed, along with myofilament calcium sensitising agents.

Toivonen HJ. Anaesthesia for patients with a transplanted organ. Acta Anaesthesiol Scand 2000; 44:812–33.
- The effects of major organ transplantation on cardiac function, respiratory function, pregnancy and immune function are reviewed, and an account of common major illnesses post-transplantation provided. Aspects of preoperative evaluation and intraoperative management of transplant recipients are dealt with in great detail.

Warner DO. Perioperative abstinence from cigarettes: physiologic and clinical consequences. Anesthesiology 2006; 104:356–67.
- More recent than the review of Zwissler (see below), this paper examines the effects (risks and mechanisms of injury) of smoking on cardiorespiratory function, wound and bone healing and nervous system function, the effects of smoking abstinence on these risks, and of nicotine replacement therapy on each of the above categories. The author concludes that any period of preoperative abstinence is of benefit, with no evidence of harm from only a brief period. Ceasing postoperatively alone is also of benefit. Current evidence suggests that nicotine replacement therapy is safe and effective in the perioperative period.

Wilson W, Taubert KA, Gewitz M. AHA guideline: Prevention of infective endocarditis. Circulation 2007; 116:1736–54.
- This consensus statement from the American Heart Association updates the previous guidelines published in 1997. They recommend that antibiotics be administered for the prevention of endocarditis in only a very limited number of procedures and cardiac conditions. As the decision regarding endocarditis prophylaxis usually defaults to the anaesthetist, this is an important change.

Woodward LJ, Kam PCA. Ankylosing spondylitis: recent developments and anaesthetic implications. Anaesthesia 2009; 64:540–8.
- The authors present a comprehensive review of the epidemiology, pathogenesis and clinical features of ankylosing spondylitis, including current management strategies. Problems of specific concern to the anaesthetist are examined, most notably airway management, regional anaesthetic techniques and management of the parturient with ankylosing spondylitis.

Zwissler B. Should smokers stop smoking preoperatively and if so, when? Curr Opin Anaesthesiol 2002; 15:53–5.

• The authors reviewed literature on the effects of smoking, and the effects on postoperative complications of smoking cessation. They concluded that a non-smoking interval of less than 8 weeks before surgery is insufficient to prevent major pulmonary complications, maybe even increasing complications in those at high risk. The reduction in carboxyhaemoglobin levels with even one day of non-smoking may, however, be of benefit. (Candidates should also be familiar with the College Policy Document PS 12 on this topic.)

Anaesthesia and specific situations

Domaingue CM. Anaesthesia for neurosurgery in the sitting position: a practical approach. Anaesth Intens Care 2005; 33(3):323–31.
• The author of this review presents advantages and disadvantages of the sitting position for posterior fossa surgery and discusses in detail the pathogenesis of venous air embolism (VAE), monitoring for its occurrence, and prevention and treatment of the complication. The same issue of this journal also presents a case series of 58 patients from the same author, in which the incidence of VAE was 43%.

Edgcombe H, Carter K, Yarrow S. Anaesthesia in the prone position. Br J Anaesth 2008; 100:165–83.
• This review aims to identify risks associated with the prone position and how they may be minimised. The authors explore cardiorespiratory changes that occur with prone positioning, and list in detail known complications (including neural, vascular, direct pressure, visceral and ophthalmic), and measures by which these may be reduced. They also discuss airway management and management of cardiac arrest in the prone position.

Gerges FJ, Kanazi GE, Jabbour-khoury SI. Anesthesia for laparoscopy: a review. J Clin Anesth 2006; 18:67–78.
• Pathophysiological changes of pneumoperitoneum in various patient positions are summarised in this review, along with a discussion of the choice of insufflated gas and gasless techniques. Both general and regional techniques and complications of laparoscopy are dealt with in detail.

Cardiac anaesthesia

Arrowsmith JE, Grocott HP, Reves JG, et al. Central nervous system complications of cardiac surgery. Br J Anaesth 2000; 84:378–93.
• The likelihood of perioperative stroke is 1–5% in this reviewed series. Perioperative cognitive dysfunction may affect up to 80% of patients undergoing cardiac surgery. Cerebral protection is discussed, as are avenues of future research.

Fergusson DA, Hebert PC, Mazer CD, et al. A comparison of aprotinin and lysine analogues in high-risk cardiac surgery. N Engl J Med 2008; 358:2319–31.
• Commonly known as the BART trial, this multicentre, randomised trial assigned 2331 high-risk cardiac surgical patients, comparing the efficacy and

mortality of aprotinin, tranexamic acid and aminocaproic acid. The aprotinin group had increased mortality compared to the lysine analogues, confirming the conclusions of the Mangano paper (listed below).

Heames RM, Gill RS, Ohri SK, et al. Off-pump coronary artery surgery. Anaesthesia 2002; 57:676–85.

- Discusses surgical and anaesthetic techniques for off-pump surgery with short-term comparisons to on-pump surgery. There is a discussion of potential advantages and a brief discussion of possible complications and disadvantages of the technique.

Mangano DT, Tudor IC, Dietzel C. The risk associated with aprotinin in cardiac surgery. N Engl J Med 2006; 354:353–65.

- The authors discuss the paradox of the use of antifibrinolytic therapy to limit blood loss in patients undergoing surgery for ST-elevation myocardial infarction despite medical treatments of fibrinolysis to limit thrombosis for the same condition. They prospectively assessed aprotinin, aminocaproic acid and tranexamic acid compared to no agent in over 4000 patients undergoing revascularisation. Only aprotinin was associated with an increased risk of adverse events, with double the risk of renal failure, 55% increase in re-infarction or heart failure and nearly double the risk of stroke or encephalopathy. Although an observational study, not a randomised controlled trial, the results led the authors to flag serious concerns about the ongoing use of aprotinin in this setting.

Skarvan K. The role of transoesophageal echocardiography for anaesthetists. Curr Opin Anaesthesiol 2000; 13:667–74.

- An early, somewhat limited review of the role of TOE for anaesthetists during cardiac bypass, valve replacement and non-cardiac surgery. Useful in its discussion of safety issues of the technique and the role of dedicated practitioner for intraoperative monitoring.

Cardiovascular risk and myocardial protection in anaesthesia

American College of Cardiology, American Heart Association. ACC/AHA 2007 guidelines on perioperative cardiovascular evaluation and care for noncardiac surgery: executive summary. Anesthesia and Analgesia 2008; 106:685–712.

- This is the most recent update of the 2002 guidelines, with formal written recommendations for preoperative patient evaluation (resting ECG, echocardiography, stress-testing) and treatment (coronary revascularisation, beta-blockers, statins, alpha-2-agonists), including intraoperative recommendations for agent use, transoesophageal echocardiography, temperature control, blood glucose control, use of pulmonary artery catheters, perioperative ST-segment monitoring and surveillance for perioperative myocardial infarction. All of these are discussed in detail and there is an extensive reference list which candidates should find helpful for further reading. One wonders if the change in format (written vs tabulated guidelines) was influenced by the article of Auerbach and Goldman (see below).

American College of Cardiology, American Heart Association. ACC/AHA guideline update on perioperative cardiovascular evaluation for noncardiac surgery. Circulation 2006; 113:2662–74.

- The first update of the 2002 guidelines, with a focus on perioperative beta-blocker therapy and review of available data.

American College of Cardiology, American Heart Association. ACC/AHA guideline update on perioperative cardiovascular evaluation for noncardiac surgery. Circulation 2002; 105:1257–67.

- This is a definitive reference on perioperative cardiac risk, and essential reading. It outlines the methodology behind the current guidelines and emphasises preoperative evaluation. Minor, intermediate and major clinical predictors of cardiovascular risk are listed. The concept of metabolic equivalents is explained in detail. Cardiac risk stratification of surgical procedures (high, intermediate and low) is given. Stepwise algorithms for assessment and further investigation are provided.

American College of Cardiology, American Heart Association, European Society of Cardiology. ACC/AHA/ESC 2006 guidelines for the management of patients with atrial fibrillation – executive summary. Circulation 2006; 114:257–354.

- These guidelines are a revision of 2001 guidelines for the assessment and management of patients with atrial fibrillation. Usefully, the collaborators provide a discussion of pathophysiological mechanisms and classification of atrial fibrillation, guidelines for patient evaluation, and recommendations on rate control, thromboembolism prophylaxis and cardioversion. Special consideration is given to atrial fibrillation in the settings of acute myocardial infarction, WPW syndrome, hyperthyroidism, pregnancy, pulmonary disease and hypertrophic obstructive cardiomyopathy.

Auerbach A, Goldman L. Assessing and reducing the cardiac risk of noncardiac surgery. Circulation 2006; 113:1361–76.

- Fascinating reading when taken in context of the above ACA guidelines, this review of evidence was written between the most recent ACA guideline updates, and highlights limitations in published evidence leading to the 2006 updated guidelines. While many recommendations are similar, the authors present alternative flowcharts for patient management.

Devereaux PJ, Yang H, Yusuf S, et al. Effects of extended-release metoprolol succinate in patients undergoing non-cardiac surgery (POISE trial): a randomised controlled trial. Lancet 2008; 371:1839–47.

- This multicentre trial enlisted over 8000 patients with known or at risk for arteriosclerotic disease to receive either metoprolol or placebo immediately preoperatively and continuing for 30 days. While fewer patients in the beta-blocker group suffered myocardial infarction, there were more deaths and more strokes in this group. This study increases awareness of risks of blanket beta-blocker therapy, and is discussed further in the editorial by Sear et al. (listed below). This is essential reading, and the topic of perioperative beta blockade is, not surprisingly, gaining popularity as an examination question.

Howard-Alpe GM, de Bono J, Hudsmith L, et al. Coronary artery stents and non-cardiac surgery. Br J Anaesth 2007; 98:560–74.
- Patients with coronary stents presenting for surgery are common in clinical practice and candidates should have a rational understanding of management options for these patients. This article discusses different types of stents (drug eluting and bare metal stents) and antiplatelet agents which are commonly used in conjunction with stents. Indications for coronary revascularisation are also tabled. The authors tackle the issue of balancing the risk of stent thrombosis against that of surgical bleeding (especially when dual antiplatelet therapy is employed) and how to assess these risks in individual patients. In general, aspirin should be continued through the perioperative period for most surgery (with the possible exceptions of intracranial and prostate surgery); options for alternative anticoagulation (when antiplatelet drugs are ceased) are discussed, including the notion that heparin alone is unlikely to protect against stent thrombosis as it has few antiplatelet properties. Issues relating to the placement and removal of neuraxial and central venous catheters are also mentioned.

Landesberg G, Mosseri M, Wolf Y, et al. Perioperative myocardial ischemia and infarction. Anesthesiology 2002; 96:264–70.
- This study monitored 185 vascular surgical patients with 12 lead ECG analysis and serial troponin measurements to determine the most sensitive combination of leads for assessing ischaemia. The authors concluded that V4 was more sensitive than V5 at detecting ischaemia, and that two or more leads were required to achieve a sensitivity of >95% for ischaemia and infarction.

London JL. New practice guidelines for perioperative beta blockade from the United States and Europe: incremental progress or a necessary evil? Can J Anesth 2010; 57:301–12.
- This recent editorial gives an outline of the controversial history of perioperative beta blockade and relates this to the latest AHA and European guidelines on the topic. The impact and shortfalls of the POISE trial are discussed in a somewhat philosophical tone.

Mangano DT, Layug EL, Wallace A, et al. Effect of atenolol on mortality and cardiovascular morbidity after noncardiac surgery. N Engl J Med 1996; 335: 1713–20.
- A landmark publication illustrating the benefits of perioperative beta-blockade in patients with coronary artery disease undergoing surgery. Nearly 200 patients were randomised to receive either atenolol or placebo. A significant reduction in mortality and morbidity at 8 months was demonstrated, with benefits still evident two years post-surgery. Although some criticism has been directed at the study design (especially with regard the treatment arms), subsequent studies have added some weight to the authors' findings.

Nathanson MH, Gajraj NM. The peri-operative management of atrial fibrillation. Anaesthesia 1998; 53:665–76.
- Discusses the aetiology, features and treatment of atrial fibrillation, the relative importance of cardioversion versus rate control for acute and chronic AF and issues of thromboembolism prevention.

Newsome LT, Kutcher MA, Royster, RL. Coronary artery stents: part I. Evolution of percutaneous coronary intervention. Anesth Analg 2008; 107:552–69.

- This is the first of a two-part review that outlines the history of percutaneous coronary procedures and the development of the bare metal and drug eluting stent. The controversies associated with the effectiveness of the drug eluting stent are discussed and the growing uncertainty regarding the appropriate antiplatelet therapy is mentioned in the final part of the paper.

Newsome LT, Weller RS, Gerancher JC, et al. Coronary artery stents: part II. Perioperative considerations and management. Anesth Analg 2008; 107:570–90.

- This is the second part of the review and principally deals with the problems associated with the coronary stent and the requirement for antiplatelet therapy. The evidence and current recommendations are clearly presented; the current trend is probably for even longer continuation of clopidogrel in these cases.

Sear JW, Giles JW, Howard-Alpe G, et al. Perioperative beta-blockade, 2008: What does POISE tell us, and was our earlier caution justified? Br J Anaesth 2008; 101: 135–8.

- The authors provide an editorial analysis of the POISE results, which do not support the introduction of perioperative beta-blockers in all patients at risk of coronary disease. For every 1000 patients treated, metoprolol may prevent 15 from suffering myocardial infarction, seven from developing atrial fibrillation and three from undergoing revascularisation. However, in excess of eight patients may die and five may suffer a stroke (in most cases, ischaemic). Patients already on beta-blockers should continue on them; patients at high risk of coronary disease almost certainly benefit from this therapy in the long term. Commencing this treatment immediately preoperatively is not supported. Beta-blockers are no longer first-line therapy in other patients with arterial hypertension. Perioperative beta-blockade should only be considered in individual cases, considering individual likely risks and benefits, and can no longer be recommended for all patients at risk of coronary disease.

Stevens RD, Burri H, Tramer MR. Pharmacologic myocardial protection in patients undergoing noncardiac surgery: a quantitative systematic review. Anesth Analg 2003; 97:623–33.

- This large, systematic, quantitative meta-analysis examines the role of pharmacological agents used for myocardial protection. Benefits of beta-blockers and alpha-2 agonists in reducing ischaemia, infarction and cardiac death are discussed. Interestingly, the analysis found little use for perioperative calcium channel antagonists or nitroglycerin in this regard.

Coagulation and anaesthesia

Gibbs NM. Point-of-care assessment of antiplatelet agents in the perioperative period: a review. Anaes Intens Care 2009; 37:354–69.

- This review assesses the strengths and weaknesses of various point-of-care platelet function assessment methods in relation to antiplatelet drug effects. The author concedes that there is no simple method of monitoring antiplatelet drugs in the perioperative period. The paper also contains useful summaries of the physiology of platelet function, the mechanism of action of antiplatelet drugs and descriptions of the various methods of platelet function assessment.

Kearon C, Hirsch J. Current concepts: management of anticoagulation before and after elective surgery. N Engl J Med 1997; 336:1506–11.
- The authors outline problems of stopping long-term warfarin therapy in the perioperative period and give a rationale for perioperative management of these patients, with emphasis on management of perioperative heparinisation.

Martlew VJ. Peri-operative management of patients with coagulation disorders. Br J Anaesth 2000; 85:445–55.
- This review gives a good overview of the haemophilias, von Willebrand's disease, platelet defects, consumptive coagulopathy, disseminated intravascular coagulation, haemolysis, thrombocytopaenia, and problems of massive transfusion, as well as coagulation defects occurring in other chronic disorders. Prophylactic unfractionated heparin and low molecular weight heparins are compared.

Vitin AA, Dembo G, Vater Y, et al. Anesthetic implications of the new anticoagulant and antiplatelet drugs. J Clin Anaesth 2008; 20:228–37.
- A concise summary of the new (and old) antiplatelet and anticoagulant drugs, including an easily understood classification system. The recommendations regarding the implications of these agents in the perioperative period are clearly presented.

Watts SA, Gibbs NM. Outpatient management of the chronically anticoagulated patient for elective surgery. Anaes Intens Care 2003; 31(2):145–54.
- Presents an easy-to-follow approach to the management of warfarin in the elective surgical patient. The guideline allows for the stratification of risk with the result that most patients can be managed safely as outpatients.

Complications and consent in anaesthesia

Borgeat A, Blumenthal S. Nerve injury and regional anaesthesia. Curr Opin Anaesthesiol 2004; 17:417–21.
- In this brief review the authors discuss the incidence of nerve injury after regional anaesthesia and examine mechanisms of neural damage, including classification of peripheral nerve injuries, the role of stretch and compression, and neurotoxicity of local anaesthetics.

Deiner S, Silverstein JH. Postoperative delirium and cognitive dysfunction. Br J Anaesth 2009; 103(suppl. I):i41–i46.
- This review defines the separate entities of postoperative delirium and cognitive dysfunction and discusses the distinguishing features, risk factors, possible aetiologies and management strategies.

Dierdorf SF. Anesthesia and informed consent. Curr Opin Anaesthesiol 2002; 15:349–50.

- Interesting comments are presented on the philosophy of informed consent in anaesthesia, including current trends. In some ways the author argues against written consent for every patient, but concedes the usefulness of a generic information form.

Dodds C, Allison J. Postoperative cognitive deficit in the elderly surgical patient. Br J Anaesth 1998; 81:449–62.
- This is a review of studies dealing with this problem, including a discussion of likely aetiologies (drugs, physiological changes, neuromodulation). It cites an incidence of up to 25%, and suggests areas of future research to reduce this figure.

Engelhardt T, Webster NR. Pulmonary aspiration of gastric contents in anaesthesia. Br J Anaesth 1999; 83:453–60.
- An evidence-based approach that considers pathophysiology, incidence, morbidity, mortality and treatment options. Overall, the incidence of the condition is very low, surprisingly also in paediatric and obstetric populations. Morbidity and mortality associated with aspiration is also very low. The authors state that there is no evidence for the use of pH-increasing or volume-reducing drugs as premedicants, and that in fact their use may be harmful.

Gan TJ, Meyer TA, Apfel CC, et al. Society for Ambulatory Anesthesia guidelines for the management of postoperative nausea and vomiting. Anesth Analg 2007; 105:1615–28.
- These guidelines were formulated from a review of the current literature from 2002 onwards, and include an analysis of the strength of evidence in each category. Patient, anaesthetic and surgical risk factors are tabulated, as are basic strategies to reduce risks (use of regional anaesthesia, avoidance of nitrous oxide and volatiles, use of propofol, minimisation of opioids and neostigmine, and adequate hydration). Antiemetic pharmacological therapy is discussed in detail, including multimodal therapy and its optimal timing, cost-effectiveness and rescue therapies.

Gosney MA. Acute confusional states and dementias: peri-operative considerations. Curr Anaesth Crit Care 2005; 16:34–9.
- This review provides a good description and definitions of delirium, dementia and psychosis and their pharmacological management. Disappointingly, despite the title, there is no indepth discussion of the problem of the acute confusional state in the immediate postoperative period (i.e. possibly caused during a period of general anaesthesia).

Grant GP, Szirth BC, Bennett HL, et al. Effects of prone and reverse Trendelenburg positioning on ocular parameters. Anesthesiology 2010; 112:57–65.
- This pilot study of awake volunteers assessed intraocular pressure, choroidal layer thickness and optic nerve diameter in the prone position over 5 hours, and showed that an increase in all of these variables is not attenuated by elevation of the head of the bed. These findings are independent of anaesthesia and fluid administration, and have implications for the potential development of ischaemic optic neuropathy in prone patients.

Gravenstein D. Transurethral resection of the prostate (TURP) syndrome: a review of the pathophysiology and management. Anesth Analg 1997; 84:438–46.

• This review provides a very detailed description of the pathophysiology of TURP syndrome and its consequences. It recommends monitoring serum osmolality, as well as sodium. Similar consequences are reported for endometrial ablation. Treatment options are discussed.

Grewal S, Hocking G, Wildsmith JAW. Epidural abscesses. Br J Anaesth 2006; 96:292–302.
• The authors of this review of the available literature since 1966 have compiled a useful summary of risk factors, pathogenesis, clinical presentation, diagnosis, management and preventative strategies for this feared complication of neuraxial block. They highlight the mathematical difficulties in estimating the true risk (somewhere between 1:1000 and 1:100,000), which would require major prospective surveillance to determine with more accuracy.

Jenkins K, Baker AB. Consent and anaesthetic risk. Anaesthetic 2003; 58(10): 962–84.
• The authors of this review have attempted to quantify common risks in anaesthesia by conducting a review of the literature from 1966 onwards. Not surprisingly, actual rates vary widely between studies and over time. However, they have constructed a table of predicted incidence of complications, including cardiac arrest, death, awareness, respiratory complications, anaphylaxis, sore throat, dental damage and peripheral nerve injury. A similar table has been constructed for predicted incidence of complications of regional anaesthesia. The authors compare risk levels to a 'community cluster logarithmic scale of risk classification', which lists risk levels of other lifetime events (risk of traffic death, winning lottery, lightning strike, etc.) and may help put risks into perspective when obtaining consent from patients.

Jones D, Story DA. Serotonin syndrome and the anaesthetist. Anaesth Intens Care 2005; 33:181–7.
• This review gives a thorough description of the pathophysiology of serotonin syndrome, including clinical features, diagnostic criteria, differential diagnoses and a list of causative agents. Management strategies and anaesthetic implications are discussed.

Kranke P, Eberhart LH, Roewer N, et al. Pharmacological treatment of postoperative shivering: a quantative systematic review of randomized controlled trials. Anesth Analg 2002; 94:453–60.
• Systematic review of pharmacological interventions for postoperative shivering, calculating relative risk and number needed to treat with the following: pethidine, clonidine, ketanserin, and doxapram, and the most effective doses of pethidine (25 mg), doxapram (100 mg) and clonidine (150 mcg) calculated (NNT = 2), as these were the most effective interventions.

McHardy FE, Chung F. Postoperative sore throat: cause, prevention and treatment. Anaesthesia 1999; 54:444–53.
• A review that examines the incidence and aetiology of sore throat with endotracheal intubation and laryngeal mask airway insertion. For endotracheal

intubation the most effective preventative strategies included careful technique, reducing tube size (to reduce area in contact with tracheal mucosa) and carefully controlling intracuff pressure. Local anaesthetic gel made the incidence worse. Insertion of a partially or fully inflated laryngeal mask was found to reduce the incidence of sore throat.

Pollard JB. Cardiac arrest during spinal anesthesia: common mechanisms and strategies for prevention. Anesth Analg 2001; 92:252–6.
- This article highlights that cardiac arrest during spinal anaesthesia is not uncommon, and not confined to subgroups of the elderly and high ASA status. They note that sympathetic blockade is two to six levels higher than sensory blockade and venous return may be impaired, the combination of which may contribute to bradycardia and cardiac arrest. Maintaining adequate preload and aggressively treating bradycardia are important preventative strategies. For severe bradycardia or actual arrest, prompt full resuscitation doses of adrenaline may improve outcome.

Rudolph T, Knudsen K. A case of fatal caffeine poisoning. Acta Anaesthesiol Scand 2010; 54:521–3.
- The authors present a case of poisoning with 10,000 mg of caffeine, ultimately resulting in death. Pharmacology and toxicology are discussed, along with a discussion of treatment options. As a guide for candidates' last-minute exam preparation, caffeine may be regarded as toxic in doses of 20 mg/kg, and >150 mg/kg may be lethal.

Ruesch S, Walder B, Tramec MR. Complications of central venous catheters: internal jugular versus subclavian access – a systematic review. Crit Care Med 2002; 30:454–60.
- Meta-analysis of over 4000 cases (no randomised trials) comparing the above. Overall, there were more arterial punctures but fewer catheter malpositions with internal jugular placement, with no difference in the incidence of haemo- or pneumothorax or vessel occlusion. The authors emphasise the need for a proper randomised trial concerning this issue.

Sawyer RJ, Richmond MN, Hickey JD, et al. Peripheral nerve injuries associated with anaesthesia. Anaesthesia 2000; 55:980–91.
- Review of the pathophysiology, aetiology and contributing factors associated with peripheral nerve injuries, including a classification of injury and the role of nerve conduction studies. Specific injuries and their prevention are discussed, as are medico-legal implications.

Thompson A, Balser JR. Perioperative cardiac arrhythmias. Br J Anaesth 2004; 93:86–94.
- This article provides a useful revision for basic physiological mechanisms of cardiac ion channels and action potential, as well as the pathophysiology of re-entry and automaticity. The authors review causes and treatment options for supraventricular and ventricular arrhythmias, including the relationship between droperidol, QT prolongation and malignant arrhythmias, and the role of pacemakers and defibrillators.

Tramer MR. A rational approach to the control of postoperative nausea and vomiting: evidence from systematic reviews. Part II. Recommendations for prevention and treatment, and research agenda. Acta Anaesthesiol Scand 2001; 45:14–19.
- A comprehensive synthesis of the recent literature on this topic, which highlights the need for systematic unbiased reviews. It draws the conclusion that monotherapy alone is unlikely to be of benefit and that treatment is more cost-effective than prevention.

Turnbull DK, Shepherd DB. Post-dural puncture headache: pathogenesis, prevention and treatment. Br J Anaesth 2003; 91:718–29.
- A useful review of the anatomy and pathophysiology of dural puncture headache, the mechanics of various needles, the incidence of the complications and a consideration of various treatment modalities and their efficacy.

Wheeler SJ, Wheeler DW. Medication errors in anaesthesia and critical care. Anaesthesia 2005; 60:257–73.
- This review looks at the problem of medication errors in the context of anaesthesia and critical care, defining slips, lapses and mistakes as distinct entities, listing the types of medication errors made, estimating incidence and exploring possible aetiologies and strategies to reduce the problem.

White SM, Baldwin TJ. Consent for anaesthesia. Anaesthesia 2003; 58:760–74.
- The authors present an argument for the provision of a standardised written consent form for anaesthesia. They review current English guidelines and put forward arguments (based on English law) supporting the use of such consent, especially to retrospectively defend a claim of negligence. Several interesting special cases are discussed.

Endocrine disease and anaesthesia

Farling PA. Thyroid disease. Br J Anaesth 2000; 85:15–28.
- A good summary of thyroid disease relevant to anaesthesia, including pathophysiology of thyroid disease and anaesthesia for thyroid surgery. Excellent photos and imaging studies are provided. Postoperative complications are also discussed in detail.

McAnulty GR, Robertshaw HJ, Hall GM. Anaesthetic management of patients with diabetes mellitus. Br J Anaesth 2000; 85:80–90.
- This review discusses diagnostic criteria, pathophysiology and current treatment options for diabetes, the challenges of perioperative management of these patients with some useful algorithms, anaesthetic techniques and perioperative complications.

Prys-Roberts C. Phaeochromocytoma – recent progress in its management. Br J Anaesth 2000; 85:44–57.
- The author discusses clinical presentation and diagnosis, important concepts in preoperative pharmacological control, and a discussion of techniques for surgery and anaesthesia, including management of complications.

Robertshaw HJ, Hall GM. Diabetes mellitus: anaesthetic management. Anaesthesia 2006; 61:1187–90.

- This paper provides a very concise (but still useful) summary of perioperative considerations for diabetic patients, including mechanisms of oral hypoglycaemic agent action, factors influencing blood glucose levels, and perioperative fluid, electrolyte and insulin management.

Smith M, Hirsch NP. Pituitary disease and anaesthesia. Br J Anaesth 2000; 85: 3–14.

- This review gives a summary of pituitary anatomy, physiology and pathophysiology, including preoperative diagnosis and management of pituitary tumours, preoperative assessment and management of patients with acromegaly and Cushing's disease and the perioperative management of anaesthesia, including postoperative treatment of diabetes insipidus and hypernatraemia.

Tasch MD. Corticosteroids and anaesthesia. Curr Opin Anaesthesiol 2002; 15:377–81.

- A review of recent articles concerning the supplementation of 'stress' steroids in the perioperative period. The authors conclude that the doses currently recommended by some are probably in excess of patient requirements. The magnitude of complications from steroid supplementation has probably also been overstated, so other benefits from current trends may be seen.

Intensive care topics

Australian and New Zealand Intensive Care Society. The ANZICS statement on death and organ donation. 3rd edn. Melbourne: ANZICS, 2008.

- These are the comprehensive Australasian guidelines for the diagnosis and management of brain death and organ donation, including useful discussions on medico-legal, ethical and family/staff welfare aspects. They should be considered essential reading for candidates.

Bugge JF. Brain death and its implications for management of the potential organ donor. Acta Anaesthesiol Scand 2009; 53:1239–50.

- This review discusses the physiological changes that occur as a result of brain death and their consequences for the transplanted organs. The rationale for current donor management strategies is discussed.

Finfer S, Chittock DR, Su SY, et al. Intensive versus conventional glucose control in critically ill patients. N Engl J Med 2009; 360:1283–97.

- Also known as the NICE-SUGAR study, this large, multicentre, randomised trial was a collaboration of the ANZICS clinical trials group and the Canadian Critical Care Trials Group. They randomised intensive care patients to either tight blood glucose control (BSL 4.5–6.0 mmol/L) or conventional blood glucose control (BSL 10.0 mmol/L or less). The tight control group was found to have a higher incidence of hypoglycaemic episodes and a higher mortality. This study has reversed the trend of increasingly tight sugar control that was suggested to be beneficial in earlier studies.

Forrest P. Anaesthesia and right ventricular failure. Anaes Intens Care 2009; 37:370–85.

- This review highlights the prevalence of right ventricular dysfunction and its aetiology and pathophysiology. Strategies to support right ventricular function and reduce pulmonary vascular resistance are discussed, including levosimendan, milrinone, iloprost and sildenafil.

Hevesi ZG, Lopukhin SY, Angelini G, et al. Supportive care after brain death for the donor candidate. Int Anesthesiol Clin 2006; 44:21–34.

- This concise review discusses the pathophysiological deterioration leading to brain death and lists clinical criteria leading to the diagnosis, along with a consideration of the therapeutic shift from cerebral protection to donor optimisation once the diagnosis of brain death is made. Management of subsequent complications is discussed in detail, including diabetes insipidus, hypotension, hypothermia, hyperglycaemia, coagulopathy and endocrine deficiency.

Mebazaa A, Karpati P, Renaud E, et al. Acute right ventricular failure – from pathophysiology to new treatments. Intens Care Med 2004; 30:185–96.

- An interesting review of the pathophysiology of right ventricular function with an appraisal of diagnosis and treatment of right ventricular failure, including the use of inhaled nitric oxide/prostacyclin, and calcium sensitising agents such as levosimendan.

Myburgh J, Cooper DJ, Finfer S, et al. Saline or albumin for fluid resuscitation in patients with traumatic brain injury. N Engl J Med 2007; 357:874–84.

- This paper was the result of a post-hoc follow-up of the SAFE study conducted by the ANZICS clinical trials group (see SAFE Study Investigators 2004 New England Journal of Medicine 350:2247–56). The original study was a randomised, multicentre, double-blind trial that showed no difference in all cause mortality in intensive care patients, whether they were resuscitated with normal saline or 4% albumin. This finding reversed the anti-colloid bias that had existed following a major meta-analysis published in the late 1990s. The post-hoc follow-up selected the group suffering traumatic brain injury, and concluded that fluid resuscitation with albumin was associated with a higher mortality than resuscitation with saline.

Monitoring and equipment in anaesthesia

Gomez CH, Palazzo MGA. Pulmonary artery catheterization in anaesthesia and intensive care. Br J Anaesth 1998; 81:945–56.

- A useful review of the use of the pulmonary artery catheter, including its insertion, pressure waveforms and their interpretation, thermodilution, continuous cardiac output and mixed venous oxygen saturation, and right ventricular function. Practicalities of its use are discussed, including indications and how it may aid patient management.

Hatfield A, Bodenham A. Ultrasound: an emerging role in anaesthesia and intensive care. Br J Anaesth 1999; 83:789–800.

- This older but interesting article discusses the physics and practicalities of ultrasound techniques, and its use in vascular access, chest drainage, echocardiography, airway evaluation and neural blockade. (Candidates are referred to the section in this chapter that deals with regional anaesthesia for modern appraisals of the concomitant use of ultrasound.)

Jhanji S, Dawson J, Pearse RM. Cardiac output monitoring: basic science and clinical application. Anaesthesia 2008; 63(2):172–81.
- Although mainly of interest to primary examination candidates, this recent review article is a clearly written and clinically relevant account of the evolution of cardiac output monitoring devices. Physiological and mathematical principles are clearly explained, and the following techniques described in detail: pulmonary artery catheter techniques, trans-pulmonary lithium- or thermo-dilution and arterial waveform analysis, oesophageal and supra-sternal Doppler, transoesophageal echocardiography, pulmonary gas clearance, electrical impedance and electrical velocimetry.

Magder S. Central venous pressure monitoring. Curr Opin Crit Care 2006; 12:219–27.
- Candidates should have a rationale for the employment of invasive monitoring. This article provides such a rationale, outlines information that can be obtained from a central venous pressure trace and gives illustrated examples of factors that can influence its measurement.

Myles PS, Leslie K, McNeil J, et al. Bispectral index monitoring to prevent awareness during anaesthesia: the B-Aware randomized controlled trial. Lancet 2004; 363:1757–63.
- The first prospective, randomised, double-blinded trial of bispectral index monitoring in 2463 patients at high risk of awareness, showing an 82% reduction in awareness with use of the device, with patients assessed immediately postoperatively, and up to 30 days. A landmark, multicentred, Australasian trial.

Sessler DI. Temperature monitoring and perioperative thermoregulation. Anesthesiology 2008; 109:318–38.
- This comprehensive account discusses thermoregulatory mechanisms, and methods and limitations of measuring core temperature. Impairment of normal thermoregulation during general and neuraxial anaesthesia is highlighted, and the author makes a recommendation that temperature be measured in all patients undergoing major surgery during regional anaesthesia, and all other surgery of greater than 1 hour's duration.

Shanewise JS, Cheung AT, Aronson S, et al. ASE/SCA guidelines of performing a comprehensive intraoperative multiplane transesophageal echocardiography examination: Recommendations of the American Society of Echocardiography Council for Intraoperative Echocardiography and the Society of Cardiovascular Anesthesiologists Task Force for Certification in Perioperative Transesophageal Echocardiography. Anesth Analg 1999; 89:870–84.
- This early consensus paper outlines the 20 basic views required in a comprehensive intraoperative TOE examination, as well as discussing the relevant cardiac anatomy and safety issues.

Torda TA. Monitoring neuromuscular transmission. Anaesth Intens Care 2002; 30:123–33.

• The author of this review provides a thought-provoking discussion on the rationale for the use and monitoring of neuromuscular blocking agents, and the methods of evaluation, with an emphasis on patterns of stimulation available and which muscular site to monitor. It highlights the hazards of incomplete reversal of paralysis and draws the conclusion that neuromuscular monitoring should be mandatory whenever paralysing agents are employed.

Muscle disorders and anaesthesia

Hopkins P. Malignant hyperthermia: advances in clinical management and diagnosis. Br J Anaesth 2000; 85:118–28.

• A useful overview of the history, diagnosis and anaesthetic associations of malignant hyperthermia. Recent laboratory advances and a discussion of molecular genetics are included.

Stevens RD. Neuromuscular disorders and anaesthesia. Curr Opin Anaesthesiol 2001; 14:693–8.

• Gives a brief overview of motor neurone disorders, Guillain-Barré peripheral neuropathy, myasthenia gravis, myasthenic syndrome, myopathies and muscular dystrophies and malignant hyperthermia. The provided references give a comprehensive coverage of the topic.

Neuroanaesthesia

Guy J, McGrath BJ, Borel CO, et al. Perioperative management of aneurysmal subarachnoid hemorrhage: part 1. Operative management. Anesth Analg 1995; 81:1060–72.

• This is the first of two reviews on this popular examination topic, and an excellent summary of the epidemiology, clinical features, classification, pathophysiology, investigation and preoperative management of subarachnoid haemorrhage. Intraoperative issues are also discussed in detail.

Hans P, Bonhomme V. Neuroprotection with anaesthetic agents. Curr Opin Anaesthesiol 2001; 14:491–6.

• An interesting review which discusses neuroprotection in terms of cellular and biochemical pathways. It discusses animal models and reviews the neuroprotective effects of anaesthetic agents, as discussed in the current literature.

Harrison FA, Mackersie A, McEwan A, et al. The sitting position for neurosurgery in children: a review of 16 years' experience. Br J Anaesth 2002; 88:12–17.

• A retrospective review of 407 cases of the sitting position in neurosurgery for children, specifically examining the incidence and consequences of venous air embolism (VAE). VAE occurred in 9.3% of cases, with significant haemodynamic consequences in 2% of all cases. All episodes responded to treatment and there was no long-term morbidity or mortality associated with its occurrence in this series.

McGrath BJ, Guy J, Borel CO, et al. Perioperative management of aneurysmal subarachnoid hemorrhage: part 2. Postoperative management. Anesth Analg 1995; 81:1295–302.
- The sequel and postoperative instalment of these reviews. Cerebral vasospasm is the focus of this article, including pathophysiology, diagnosis, prevention and management. Other complications, such as hydrocephalus, seizures, hyponatraemia and neurogenic pulmonary oedema, are dealt with briefly.

Priebe HJ. Aneurysmal subarachnoid haemorrhage and the anaesthetist. Br J Anaesth 2007; 99:102–18.
- This fairly extensive review of the topic outlines the features of subarachnoid haemorrhage that are of importance to the anaesthetist, including aetiology, pathophysiology, classification systems and diagnosis. A detailed discussion on the anaesthetic management of clipping and coiling procedures is included. There is also a good description of the complications of subarachnoid haemorrhage with emphasis on the management of vasospasm.

Raw DA, Beattie JK, Hunter JM. Anaesthesia for spinal surgery in adults. Br J Anaesth 2003; 91:886–904.
- This review discusses the conditions requiring major spinal surgery and the likely co-morbidities that may be encountered. Anaesthetic considerations, such as airway management, positioning, blood loss, pain management and spinal cord monitoring, are examined in detail.

Obstetric anaesthesia

Cox PBW, Gogarten W, Marcus MAE. Maternal cardiac disease. Curr Opin Anaesthesiol 2005; 18:257–62.
- This review examines normal physiological changes in pregnancy and the impact of concomitant cardiovascular disease, including acute coronary syndromes, peripartum cardiomyopathy, hypertrophic obstructive cardiomyopathy, cardiac valve stenoses, congenital heart defects and Marfan's syndrome. Consideration of fetal and maternal risks in the management of these is discussed.

Duffy PJ, Crosby ET. The epidural blood patch. Resolving the controversies. Can J Anaesth 1999; 46:878–86.
- A review of case series and comparative studies of epidural blood patching for post-dural puncture headache. Interestingly, analysis shows that the treatment is less efficacious than previously thought, with relief in 61–75% on initial patch. Patching with non-blood solution results in a higher recurrence rate of headache. Prophylactic injection of saline or blood decreases the incidence of headache.

Duley L, Magpie Trial Collaborative Group. Do women with pre-eclampsia, and their babies, benefit from magnesium sulphate? The Magpie Trial: a randomised placebo-controlled trial. Lancet 2002; 359:1877–90.

- This landmark, randomised, controlled trial allocated over 10,000 eligible pre-eclamptic women to receive either magnesium sulphate or a placebo. Those in the treatment arm had a 58% lower risk of eclampsia, and maternal mortality was also lower (relative risk 0.55). There was no statistically significant difference in neonatal outcome.

Kuczkowski KM. Post-dural puncture headache in the obstetric patient: an old problem. New solutions. Minerva Anestesiol 2004; 70:823–30.
- This review gives a historical perspective on the problem of dural puncture and the pathophysiology of meninges and cerebrospinal fluid. They describe symptomatology and current treatment modalities (including caffeine, sumatriptan, epidural saline, epidural dextran, subarachnoid catheters and epidural blood patch). The authors then propose a five-point protocol for preventing headache when the dura is punctured: re-injecting any CSF in the syringe, passing catheter into subarachnoid space, injecting 5 mL saline through catheter, continuing analgesia via catheter and leaving the catheter in situ for 12–20 hours. They conclude that further studies are needed to determine the effectiveness of the protocol.

Lee A, Ngan Kee WD, Gin T. A quantitative, systematic review of randomized controlled trials of ephedrine versus phenylephrine for the management of hypotension during spinal anesthesia for Cesarean delivery. Anesth Analg 2002; 94:920–6.
- One of several recent articles examining this issue, these authors conducted a meta-analysis of randomised, controlled trials comparing ephedrine and phenylephrine in both the prevention and the treatment of maternal hypotension. The authors conclude that ephedrine should no longer be regarded as the treatment of choice; phenylephrine showed higher umbilical arterial pH values but (not surprisingly) an increase in maternal bradycardia. There was no difference between the drugs in the success of management of hypotension.

Pan PH, D'Angelo R. Anesthetic and analgesic management of mitral stenosis during pregnancy. Reg Anesth Pain Med 2004; 29:610–15.
- The authors conducted a literature review to determine the best labour, Caesarean and perioperative management of parturients with mitral stenosis. Not surprisingly, the total number of articles was small (mostly level III and IV evidence studies), owing to the increasingly rare nature of the disease. Two original case reports are also provided, describing both neuraxial and general anaesthetic techniques for management of emergency delivery. Anti-arrhythmic and anticoagulant issues are also outlined.

Ray P, Murphy GJ, Shutt LE. Recognition and management of maternal cardiac disease in pregnancy. Br J Anaesth 2004; 93:428–39.
- This is a very good overview of incipient (peripartum cardiomyopathy, aortic dissection and myocardial infarction) and chronic (congenital heart disease, pulmonary hypertension, valvular heart disease and transplantation) maternal cardiac problems. Individual descriptions of the relevant problems and diagnostic and management recommendations for each are provided.

Roberts JM, Cooper, DW. Pathogenesis and genetics of pre-eclampsia. Lancet 2001; 357:53–6.
- A brief but interesting article that pushes a possible genetic predisposition towards pre-eclampsia into the limelight, suggesting future avenues of research on this topic. Current thinking into pathogenetic mechanisms is also discussed.

Saravanakumar K, Rao SG, Cooper CM. Obesity and obstetric anaesthesia. Anaesthesia 2006; 61:36–48.
- This review describes the specific problems and increased anaesthetic risks associated with the combination of obesity and pregnancy in system subheadings, and tackles issues related to both regional analgesia and anaesthesia and general anaesthesia for Caesarean section. The authors suggest that placement of an epidural catheter prophylactically in labour may decrease maternal and neonatal complications associated with emergency situations.

Vercauteren M, Palit S, Soetens F, et al. Anaesthesiological considerations on tocolytic and uterotonic therapy in obstetrics. Acta Anaesthesiol Scand 2009; 53:701–9.
- The authors of this review describe the pharmacology of commonly encountered substances with uterine activity, examining in detail complications that may be associated with their use.

Ophthalmic anaesthesia

Hamilton RC. Techniques of orbital regional anaesthesia. Br J Anaesth 1995; 75:88–92.
- Describes patient assessment and choice of needle, with discussion of retrobulbar, peribulbar, sub-Tenon, perilimbal and topical blockade. References are provided for further reading on each of these techniques.

Johnson RW. Anatomy for ophthalmic anaesthesia. Br J Anaesth 1995; 75:80–7.
- This is an excellent, detailed description of all aspects of orbital anatomy relevant to anaesthesia for eye surgery. It considers the relations of the bony orbit, the globe and supporting structures, extraocular muscles, nerves, vessels and lacrimal apparatus.

Kumar CM, Williamson W, Manickham B. A review of sub-Tenon's block: current practice and recent development. Eur J Anaesthesiol 2005; 22:567–77.
- This article describes the technique of sub-Tenon block and compares it to akinetic needle techniques. The description of orbital anatomy is succinct, and the technique itself is comprehensively discussed.

Orthopaedic anaesthesia

Donaldson AJ, Thomson HE, Harper NJ, et al. Bone cement implantation syndrome. Br J Anaesth 2009; 102:12–22.

- This very good review aims to consolidate current knowledge of problems associated with cemented bone surgery. They describe a severity classification, likely incidence and clinical features, with an extensive examination of aetiologies and pathophysiology. They also identify patient, surgical and anaesthetic risk factors and methods that may reduce such risks.

Gibson PRJ. Anaesthesia for correction of scoliosis in children. Anaesth Intens Care 2004; 32:548–59.

- This review gives an excellent classification of the aetiology and pathophysiology of scoliosis, indications for surgery and surgical techniques. Preoperative patient assessment is dealt with in detail, and there is comprehensive discussion of methods of spinal cord monitoring, blood loss and coagulopathy, air embolism and other complications. Protocols for postoperative analgesic regimens are also provided.

Paediatric anaesthesia

Alalami AA, Ayoub CM, Baraka AS. Laryngospasm: review of different prevention and treatment modalities. Pediatr Anesth 2008; 18:281–8.

- This review provides a useful summary of mechanisms and risks for laryngospasm in children, including a differential diagnosis, listing methods for prevention and treatment (some of which are questionable, e.g. inhalation of 5% carbon dioxide or inducing periosteal pain of the styloid process). Conventional management algorithms are also provided.

Courtman SP, Mumby D. Children with learning disabilities. Pediatr Anesth 2008; 18:198–207.

- The authors of this review highlight the challenges faced when dealing with children with learning disabilities (reduced IQ and accompanying loss of function) in the hospital setting. Definitions, aetiologies and clinical features are listed, along with an extensive discussion of perioperative management strategies to better deal with the special requirements of these patients.

Cunliffe M, Roberts SA. Pain management in children. Curr Anaesth Crit Care 2004; 15:272–83.

- Methods for assessing pain in pre-verbal and older children are briefly discussed, along with pharmacokinetics and pharmacodynamics of commonly used analgesics. Day case analgesia, topical EMLA/amethocaine, local anaesthetic blocks and caudal analgesia are examined, along with techniques of opioid infusion, patient- and nurse-controlled analgesia and epidural infusions. Non-pharmacological methods of pain control are included, along with the specific problems of procedural analgesia and chronic pain in children.

Krauss B, Green SM. Procedural sedation and analgesia in children. Lancet 2006; 367:766–80.

- This is an extremely detailed review of literature since 1980 dealing with problems and techniques of procedural sedation in children, including pre-procedure assessment, equipment and monitoring and pharmacology of commonly used agents. Some consideration is also given to controversies in levels of practitioner skills and practice standards.

McEwan AI, Birch M, Bingham R. The preoperative management of the child with a heart murmur. Pediatr Anesth 1995; 5:151–6.
- This is an old paper, but it represents a practical approach to dealing with the child who presents for elective surgery and is discovered to have a heart murmur. Although the antibiotic guidelines are superseded, the rationale presented for deferring and investigating versus proceeding with surgery remains sensible and pragmatic.

Morton NS. Prevention and control of pain in children. Br J Anaesth 1999; 83:118–29.
- One of several useful reviews in this edition of this journal. Discusses the assessment of pain in children of different age groups, topical anaesthesia, wound infiltration, nitrous oxide and non-drug techniques (as simple measures), peripheral nerve and central neuraxial blockade (continuous and intermittent techniques), parenteral opioid techniques (including PCA and NCA). Management of complications is also discussed.

Murat I, Dubois M-C. Perioperative fluid therapy in pediatrics. Pediatr Anesth 2008; 18:363–70.
- The authors provide a rational basis for calculating daily fluid requirements, estimating preoperative fluid deficit and giving fasting guidelines for elective surgery. Intraoperative fluid management and blood glucose management is dealt with in a similar manner. Controversies relating to fluid composition and volume are also discussed.

Tait AR, Malviya S. Anesthesia for the child with an upper respiratory tract infection: still a dilemma? Anesth Analg 2005; 100:59–65.
- This article examines the decision of whether to proceed with elective surgery or not in a child who presents with an upper respiratory infection. The authors discuss the pathophysiology and potential complications associated with the majority of upper respiratory infections and formulate an algorithm for clinical decision-making. When postponed, the authors advocate 4 weeks as a prudent length of time to wait for surgery. They also discuss anaesthetic management strategies should the case proceed.

Walker SM. Pain in children: recent advances and ongoing challenges. Br J Anaesth 2008; 101:101–10.
- This recent review uses an evidence-based approach to evaluate analgesic trials in children, along with a discussion of pain assessment in neonates, developmental neurobiology and pharmacology, and the implications of the development of chronic pain in children.

Wongprasartsuk P, Stevens J. Cerebral palsy and anaesthesia. Pediatr Anesth 2002;12:296–303.
- This review provides aetiology, risk factors and a classification of cerebral palsy, along with a discussion of pharmacological therapies. Preoperative assessment and perioperative management are examined in detail, and the specific scenarios of inguinal hernia repair, antireflux surgery and scoliosis surgery are highlighted.

Pain management

Bennetto L, Patel NK, Fuller G. Trigeminal neuralgia and its management. BMJ 2007; 334:201–5.
- This overview of the condition is written in a casual style, but has useful diagrams, tables of differential diagnoses, diagnostic criteria and a discussion of causes, investigations and treatments.

Elia N, Lysakowski C, Tramer MR. Does multimodal analgesia with acetaminophen, nonsteroidal anti-inflammatory drugs, or selective cyclooxygenase-2 inhibitors and patient-controlled analgesia morphine offer advantages over morphine alone? Meta-analyses of randomized trials. Anesthesiology 2005; 103:1296–304.
- This study analysed 52 randomised controlled trials (of nearly 5000 adults), showing a decrease in morphine consumption with all regimens. Pain intensity and nausea and vomiting were reduced with non-steroidal anti-inflammatory agents, but this group showed an increased risk of severe bleeding. Selective COX-2 inhibitors were shown to increase the risk of renal failure in cardiac patients.

Hocking G, Cousins MJ. Ketamine in chronic pain management: an evidence-based review. Anesth Analg 2003; 97:1730–9.
- A comprehensive review of articles discussing the use of ketamine in chronic pain, with an evidence-based approach. The paucity of good data on the efficacy of ketamine is highlighted. The authors found no strong evidence base supporting the use of ketamine in chronic pain. Due to the incidence of side effects it is unlikely to be included in first-line treatment. In cases where ketamine is considered, the authors propose an algorithm for its use.

Mehta V, Langford RM. Acute pain management for opioid dependent patients. Anaesthesia 2006; 61:269–76.
- This very useful article defines the concepts of addiction, tolerance and physical dependence, and examines the underlying pathophysiological mechanisms of these. Useful guidelines are provided for the management of acute pain in these patients including multimodal therapies, rational use of opioids, PCA and opioid rotation techniques.

Nurmikko TJ, Eldridge PR. Trigeminal neuralgia – pathophysiology, diagnosis and current treatment. Br J Anaesth 2001; 87:117–32.
- This provides a detailed coverage of the diagnosis, differential diagnosis, pathophysiology, investigations and treatment of trigeminal neuralgia, with a review of contemporary studies. A rationale for treatment options is given.

Raja SN, Brabow TS. Complex regional pain syndrome I (reflex sympathetic dystrophy). Anesthesiology 2002; 96:1254–60.
- These authors give a review of the terminology, epidemiology and detailed discussion of the clinical features of CRPS I. A summary of the diagnosis and multimodal management follows. An excellent summary of the condition.

Remy C, Marret E, Bonnet F. State of the art of paracetamol in acute pain therapy. Curr Opin Anaesthesiol 2006; 19:562–5.

- This brief review discusses new theories of mechanisms of action of paracetamol, the need for adequate dosing, efficacy and drug interactions. There is not yet reliable evidence that addition of paracetamol to morphine regimens significantly reduces morphine side effects.

Rho RH, Brewer RP, Lamer TJ, et al. Complex regional pain syndrome. Mayo Clin Proc 2002; 77:174–80.
- This very good, concise review summarises the signs and symptoms, diagnostic tests, management strategies and treatment options for complex regional pain syndrome types 1 and 2.

Wheatley RG, Schug SA, Watson D. Safety and efficacy of postoperative epidural analgesia. Br J Anaesth 2001; 87:47–61.
- Review of the literature with evidence-based analysis of benefits and adverse outcomes associated with epidural analgesia. A protocol for its safe use postoperatively is given. The article stresses the role of the acute pain service in identifying and rapidly dealing with complications that may arise.

Pharmacology and anaesthesia

Caldwell JE, Miller RD. Clinical implications of sugammadex. Anaesthesia 2009; 64(S1):66–72.
- This interesting review deals only briefly with the clinical pharmacology of sugammadex, but instead examines the ways in which its availability may change clinical practice with respect to the use of neuromuscular blocking agents. Advantages and disadvantages are discussed, along with implications for the use or discontinuation of non-steroid muscle relaxants, and the role for neuromuscular monitoring.

Campagna JA, Forman SA. Mechanisms of action of inhaled anesthetics. N Engl J Med 2003; 348:2110–24.
- This article provides an easily read account of proposed mechanisms of anaesthetic action with an emphasis on molecular sites and ion channels, which may be of interest.

Chun R, Orser BA, Madan M. Platelet glycoprotein IIb/IIIa inhibitors: overview and implications for the anesthesiologist. Anesth Analg 2002; 95:879–88.
- One of several recent review articles on this topic. Discusses the role of glycoproteins in plaque rupture and platelet inhibitor pharmacology (abciximab, eptifibatide and tirofiban). Recent clinical studies are summarised. The authors discuss complications, including bleeding and thrombocytopenia, and issues of relevance to anaesthesia, including the timing of surgery.

Craven R. Ketamine. Anaesthesia 2007; 62:48–53.
- After a concise discussion of its pharmacological properties, the author gives some practical examples of the usefulness and versatility of ketamine with clinical examples covering the spectrum of general anaesthesia, paediatric sedation, oral usage for repeat procedures, postoperative analgesia, asthma and chronic pain.

Fawcett WJ, Haxby EJ, Male DA. Magnesium: physiology and pharmacology. Br J Anaesth 1999; 83:302–20.
- This is a detailed review of the physiology and therapeutic uses of magnesium, including its use in obstetrics, cardiology and critical care.

Gupta A, Stierer T, Zuckerman R, et al. Comparison of recovery profile after ambulatory anesthesia with propofol, isoflurane, sevoflurane and desflurane: a systematic review. Anesth Analg 2004; 98:632–41.
- The authors conducted a meta-analysis of randomised trials and compared each of the above anaesthetic agents with the others in terms of recovery profiles and side effects. Early recovery was faster with desflurane compared with propofol and isoflurane, and with sevoflurane compared with isoflurane. No major differences were found with home readiness. The incidence of side effects, especially nausea and vomiting, was less with propofol.

Himmelseher S, Durieux ME. Ketamine for perioperative pain management. Anesthesiology 2005; 102:211–20.
- The role of ketamine as an analgesic is discussed in detail, including cellular mechanisms of action and clinical uses, including combined opioid and ketamine PCA techniques, and neuraxial ketamine use.

Kam PCA, Nethery CM. The thienopyridine derivatives (platelet adenosine diphosphate receptor antagonists), pharmacology and clinical developments. Anaesthesia 2003; 58:28–35.
- A review of ticlopidine and clopidogrel, which may be encountered more commonly in clinical practice than the glycoprotein inhibitors. The authors discuss the pathophysiology of atherosclerosis and thrombosis, and the pharmacology and side effects of thienopyridines. Anaesthetic considerations are mentioned, including cessation prior to surgery.

Kam PCA, See AUL. Cyclo-oxygenase isoenzymes: physiological and pharmacological role. Anaesthesia 2000; 55:442–9.
- A very detailed account of the physiology of prostaglandins and cyclooxygenase isoforms, and the pharmacology of selective COX-2 inhibitors. This was published prior to controversies that arose surrounding the increased cardiovascular mortality in patients taking selected members of this group.

Kong VKF, Irwin MG. Gabapentin: a multimodal perioperative drug? Br J Anaesth 2007; 99:775–86.
- This review summarises the pharmacology and anti-nociceptive mechanisms of gabapentin, and also looks at clinical trial data relating to its role as part of multimodal postoperative analgesia. Newer roles in attenuating haemodynamic responses and preventing nausea and vomiting are examined briefly.

Krause T, Gerbershagen MU, Fiege M, et al. Dantrolene – a review of its pharmacology, therapeutic use and new developments. Anaesthesia 2004; 59:364–73.
- The history and pharmacology of dantrolene is described in this review, including a discussion of its side effects and drug interactions. Its therapeutic uses are outlined, including in malignant hyperthermia, neuroleptic malignant syndrome, motor spasticity, ecstasy intoxication and heat stroke.

Myles PS, Leslie K, Chan MTV, et al. ENIGMA Trial Group: Avoidance of nitrous oxide for patients undergoing major surgery: a randomized controlled trial. Anesthesiology 2007; 107:221–31.

- The ENIGMA trial comprised recruitment of over 2000 eligible patients across 19 centres. Patients undergoing surgery of at least 2 hours' duration received 70% nitrous oxide or nitrous oxide-free anaesthesia. There was no difference between groups in the primary end-point of duration of hospital stay. Examination of secondary end-points (duration of intensive care stay and complications within 30 days, including cardiorespiratory complications, awareness, thromboembolism, stroke and death) showed a lower incidence of severe nausea and vomiting, fever, wound infection and atelectasis in the nitrous-free group. The differences were attributable to either an avoidance of the toxic effects of nitrous oxide or an increase in concentration of supplemental oxygen. The authors conclude that the routine use of nitrous oxide in such patients should be questioned.

Myles PS, Leslie K, Silbert B, et al. A review of the risks and benefits of nitrous oxide in current anaesthetic practice. Anaesth Intens Care 2004; 32:165–72.

- This interesting review provided the backdrop for the ENIGMA study, and gives a comprehensive description of the side effects of nitrous oxide contrasted with the perceived benefits, raising the question of whether its use is still justified, and introducing the idea of the need for a large, randomised, controlled trial.

Oscier CD, Milner QJW. Peri-operative use of paracetamol. Anaesthesia 2009; 64:65–72.

- This review examines the pharmacology of paracetamol, including potential mechanisms of action, efficacy and routes of administration. They discuss in detail the usefulness of providing a loading dose to achieve more effective postoperative analgesia.

Regional anaesthesia

Borgeat A, Ekatodramis G, Kalberer F, et al. Acute and nonacute complications associated with interscalene block and shoulder surgery. A prospective study. Anesthesiology 2001; 95:875–80.

- Study and follow-up of 520 patients receiving standardised interscalene block for shoulder surgery, 234 of whom had an indwelling interscalene catheter. Patients were reviewed daily for 10 days, then at regular intervals to 9 months. Complications included pneumothorax and CNS toxicity. At 10 days 14% of patients had residual sensory symptoms, 8% at one month, and one patient at 9 months. Diagnoses included carpal tunnel syndrome, complex regional pain syndrome, sulcus ulnaris syndrome and plexus neuropathy/damage. There was no significant difference between the two groups (single-shot versus catheter).

Cook TM, Counsell D, Wildsmith JAW. Major complications of central neuraxial block: report on the Third National Audit Project of the Royal College of Anaesthetists. Br J Anaesth 2009; 102:179–90.

• The audit project conducted a census of over 700,000 central neuraxial blocks, and then identified 52 which met inclusion criteria for major complications. The incidence of permanent injury due to central blockade was estimated at between 2.0 and 4.2 per 100,000 cases. The incidence of paraplegia or death was estimated at between 0.7 and 1.8 per 100,000 cases.

Fowler SJ, Symons J, Sabato S, et al. Epidural analgesia compared with peripheral nerve blockade after major knee surgery: a systematic review and meta-analysis of randomized trials. Br J Anaesth 2008; 100:154–64.

• The authors conducted an analysis resulting in the inclusion of eight studies involving 464 patients undergoing knee replacement who received analgesia from either epidural or peripheral nerve block (femoral, sciatic or lumbar plexus) techniques. There was no significant difference in pain scores, nausea and vomiting or morphine consumption between the groups, but the epidural group demonstrated more frequent hypotension and urinary retention than in the peripheral block group. The authors conclude that peripheral nerve blockade provides comparable analgesia to that of epidural block, but with an improved side-effect profile and avoiding severe neuraxial complications.

Horlocker TT, Wedel DJ, Benzon H, et al. Regional anesthesia in the anticoagulated patient: defining the risks (the second ASRA Consensus Conference on Neuraxial Anesthesia and Anticoagulation). Reg Anesth Pain Med 2003; 28:172–97.

• This article represents consensus statements based on available evidence of the time. It lists recommendations for thromboembolism prophylaxis and treatment and the risk of bleeding associated with antithrombotic and thrombolytic therapy, including the incidence and outcomes of neuraxial haematoma. Fibrinolytic therapy, unfractionated and low molecular weight heparin, oral anticoagulant, antiplatelet agents and newer medications are dealt with in turn, and recommendations on the conduct and timing of major regional anaesthetic interventions put forward for each of these.

Koscielniak-Nielsen ZJ. Ultrasound-guided peripheral nerve blocks: what are the benefits? Acta Anaesthesiol Scand 2008; 52:727–37.

• The author conducted a survey of articles related to use of ultrasound for peripheral nerve blockade. There appears to be no benefit in concomitant use of electrical nerve stimulation, block performance times are reduced and dose reduction of local anaesthesia may be achieved. There was no difference in the incidence of short-duration postoperative neuropraxias when ultrasound was used. Data on the incidence of vascular complications was conflicting among the studies examined.

Neal JM, Gerancher JC, Hebl JR, et al. Upper extremity regional anesthesia: essentials of our current understanding, 2008. Reg Anesth Pain Med 2009; 34:134–70.

• This is an excellent and extremely detailed account of brachial plexus anatomy and blockade techniques, which also compares single-shot and continuous techniques. There are many anatomical photos and diagrams. Other technical aspects, such as nerve stimulation and ultrasound guidance, are examined. Local anaesthetic and adjuvant medication pharmacology are detailed, and an extensive section on block complications and their prevention is provided.

Rigg JRA, Jamrozik K, Myles PS, et al. (The MASTER Anaesthesia Trial Study Group.) Epidural anaesthesia and analgesia and outcome of major surgery: a randomised trial. Lancet 2002; 359:1276–82.

- In this trial, 915 patients with major co-morbidities were randomised into GA + epidural versus control. End point was mortality or major morbidity at 30 days. Of morbid endpoints, there was a lower incidence of respiratory failure in the epidural group, otherwise there was no difference. While no major reduction in most morbidities or mortality was demonstrated from epidural use, significantly better pain management was achieved in this group.

Rowlingson JC, Hanson PB. Neuraxial anesthesia and low-molecular-weight heparin prophylaxis in major orthopedic surgery in the wake of the latest American Society of Regional Anesthesia guidelines. Anesth Analg 2005; 100:1482–8.

- The authors review the ASRA guidelines and highlight the principles of management of timing of neuraxial/plexus anaesthesia and/or catheter removal, highlighting the relevant safety concerns.

Sites BD, Spence BC, Gallagher J, et al. Regional anesthesia meets ultrasound: a specialty in transition. Acta Anaesthesiol Scand 2008; 52:456–66.

- The authors discuss variability of neurovascular anatomy as a reason for failure of regional anaesthesia and as the source of some common complications and potential pitfalls in the use of nerve stimulators; both of these are an argument for ultrasound-guided blocks. Principles of ultrasound-guided nerve blockade are outlined, along with potential pitfalls and cost-effectiveness.

Wu CL. Regional anesthesia and anticoagulation. J Clin Anesth 2001; 13:49–58.

- A useful and detailed summary of anticoagulants in current practice, with reference to major regional anaesthetic techniques and the management thereof, including timing of agent cessation with neuraxial blockade and epidural catheter removal.

Remote locations and anaesthesia

Ding Z, White PF. Anesthesia for electroconvulsive therapy. Anesth Analg 2002; 94:1351–64.

- Comprehensive review article that describes the physiological responses to ECT, factors that modulate seizure duration, pharmacology of commonly used agents, anaesthetic techniques, problems of specific patient subpopulations (including those with intracerebral pathology, cardiovascular disease, pregnancy and neuroleptic malignant syndrome susceptibility).

Osborn IP. Magnetic resonance imaging anesthesia: new challenges and techniques. Curr Opin Anaesthesiol 2002; 15:443–8.

- Briefly considers the challenges posed by anaesthesia for MRI, then outlines techniques for the sedation or anaesthesia of children and adults, and specific issues in MRI for critical care patients.

Thoracic anaesthesia

Campos JH. Current techniques for perioperative lung isolation in adults. Anesthesiology 2002; 97:1295–301.
- This is an excellent dissertation on selection and placement of double-lumen tubes, bronchial blockers and Univent tubes, including complications.

Hillier J, Gillbe C. Anaesthesia for lung volume reduction surgery. Anaesthesia 2003; 58:1210–19.
- This review details the pathophysiology of emphysema and the rationale for surgery, surgical techniques, patient selection, anaesthetic techniques and postoperative management for this still-controversial technique.

Karzai W, Schwarzkopf K. Hypoxemia during one-lung ventilation: prediction, prevention, and treatment. Anesthesiology 2009; 110:1402–11.
- Mechanisms of hypoxia during one-lung ventilation are briefly discussed in this article, and preventative strategies (improving preoperative lung function, monitoring lung separation, ventilation strategies, oxygen administration and type of anaesthesia) are detailed. A simple, sensible approach to treatment of hypoxia during one-lung ventilation is put forward.

Slinger PD, Johnston MR. Preoperative assessment for pulmonary resection. Anesthesiol Clin N Amer 2001; 19:411–33.
- Discusses the perioperative complications associated with pulmonary surgery, and techniques for the assessment of respiratory function, including scintigraphy, spirometry, split lung function, flow–volume loops. Consideration is also given to co-existent disease.

Transfusion medicine

Barrett NA, Kam PCA. Transfusion-related acute lung injury: a literature review. Anaesthesia 2006; 61:777–85.
- The authors note the under-diagnosis and lack of awareness of this complication of blood product transfusion, and the estimates of incidence with different blood products are provided. Mechanism theories, the spectrum of clinical features, management, prognosis and prevention are all discussed in turn.

Chappell D, Jacob M, Hofmann-Kiefer K, et al. A rational approach to perioperative fluid management. Anesthesiology 2008; 109:723–40.
- An entertaining and thought-provoking essay that critically challenges many commonly held views and practices pertaining to perioperative fluid use, which, in the authors' opinion, lead to over-replacement of fluid, hypervolaemia, interstitial flooding and vascular endothelial destruction. They question the

effect of fasting on blood volume, the existence of a fluid-consuming third space and the commonly perceived magnitude of insensible losses. The authors include a detailed discussion of physiological effects of infusion of crystalloids and colloids, and propose the use of crystalloid to replace urinary and insensible losses, and colloid to replace acute blood loss or protein-rich shifts towards the interstitial space, using a protocol-based approach.

Grocott MPW, Mythen MG, Gan TJ. Perioperative fluid management and clinical outcomes in adults. Anesth Analg 2005; 100:1093–106.
- This review contains an extensive revision of fluid compartment physiology and detailed analysis of composition of various crystalloids and colloids. The authors give an account of strategies of fluid administration and rationales for intravascular volume measurements.

Shaz BH, Dente CJ, Harris RS, et al. Transfusion management of trauma patients. Anesth Analg 2009; 108:1760–8.
- This review provides definitions of massive transfusion and deals extensively with the topic of trauma-induced coagulopathy. They provide a protocol for component replacement therapy, supporting the use of a plasma:erythrocyte:platelet ratio of 1:1:1.

Spahn DR, Casutt M. Eliminating blood transfusions: new aspects and perspectives. Anaesthesiology 2000; 93:242–55.
- Complications of allogenic blood transfusion are detailed, and alternative strategies discussed: autologous donation, erythropoietin, normovolaemic haemodilution, cell salvage, artificial O_2 carriers, as well as more general strategies for surgery and anaesthesia.

Vascular anaesthesia

GALA Trial Collaborative Group. General anaesthesia versus local anaesthesia for carotid surgery (GALA): a multicentre, randomised controlled trial. Lancet 2008; 372:2132–42.
- This multicentre, randomised, controlled trial of 3526 patients compared local and general anaesthesia for carotid endarterectomy, with endpoints of stroke, myocardial infarction and death. The study was not able to detect a difference in outcome between the two groups and concluded that the technique used should be an individual decision by the surgeon and the anaesthetist in consultation with the patient.

Gelman S. The pathophysiology of aortic cross-clamping and unclamping. Anesthesiology 1995; 82:1026–57.
- A very detailed article on the physiological consequences of aortic clamping and unclamping on all of the body's organ systems. A useful reference for those with an interest in vascular anaesthesia.

Jellish WS, Seikh T, Baker WH, et al. Hemodynamic stability, myocardial ischemia, and perioperative outcome after carotid surgery with remifentanil/propofol or isoflurane/fentanyl anesthesia. J Neurosurg Anesthesiol 2003; 15:176–84.

• Sixty patients were randomised to receive either treatment. The only differences between the groups were an increased incidence of intraoperative regional wall motion abnormalities on TOE in the volatile group, and nine times the overall cost of the technique for the remifentanil group. The authors concluded that the increase in cost could not be justified on the basis of morbidity alone.

Stoneham MD, Thompson JP. Arterial pressure management and carotid endarterectomy. Br J Anaesth 2009; 102:442–52.
• This useful review discusses perioperative risk factors in patients undergoing endarterectomy and issues related to hypertension, including cerebral hyperperfusion. The authors discuss causes of haemodynamic instability intraoperatively and suggest extensive strategies for managing arterial pressure.

Swaminathan M, Stafford-Smith M. Renal dysfunction after vascular surgery. Curr Opin Anaesthesiol 2003; 16:45–51.
• This review discusses the incidence and factors associated with renal impairment and vascular surgery. Strategies for prevention are outlined, and the lack of a truly protective pharmacological agent highlighted.

Wallenborn J, Thieme V, Hertel-Gilch G, et al. Effects of clonidine and superficial cervical plexus block on hemodynamic stability after carotid endarterectomy. J Cardiothor Vasc Anesth 2008; 22:84–9.
• In this prospective observational study, 275 patients underwent general anaesthesia for carotid endarterectomy. Of these, 85 received supplemental clonidine 3 ug/kg before the end of the procedure, and 140 patients received clonidine and a superficial cervical plexus block with 20 mL 0.5% ropivacaine before induction. Both groups receiving clonidine showed significantly better haemodynamic stability postoperatively, as measured by the need for rescue medication and arterial blood pressure measurements.

Index

Page numbers followed by 'f' denote figures; those followed by 't' denote tables

Ingram Content Group UK Ltd.
Milton Keynes UK
UKHW030259170323
418721UK00008B/189